AARON'S ROD

God and mental health

John Gordon

Published on Amazon by Philadelphia Books

https://mentalhealthandgod.org

ISBN 978-0-9570970-7-0

Blessed are the poor in spirit,
for theirs is the kingdom of heaven.
(Matthew 5:3.)

CONTENTS

PREFACE

The purpose of this book is to bring hope to people suffering mental illness.

It is not for people who want treatment. Rather, it is a book for people seeking Christian spiritual healing.

It includes God, and provides a Christian understanding.

The book describes how God's healing is available for all sorts of mental distress, and how sense can be made of madness. It is offered as a result of much experience not conformed to this world (as in Romans 12:2).

Mental illness is seen to be a spiritual condition. The healing is with Messiah Jesus. That there is no room for Him in psychiatric units is a tragedy of enormous proportions.

There is too much grumbling against God, too much unbelief, and too much cynicism about what He can do. That is the road to death (see Numbers 17). But Jesus Christ overcame death. He offers eternal new life.

The only begotten Son of God, Jesus Christ, paid the price with His very lifeblood to redeem and save all people (2 Corinthians 5:15). Salvation includes healing. It includes soundness of mind. Jesus rose from the dead. Death could not hold Him. He overcame all the powers of this world, of Satan, and of death. Now he is with the Father in heaven; but He sends His Spirit to those who take hold of Him in repentance, recognizing who He is, forgiving others, accepting the victory He won, and placing their trust in Him. This way, His presence is with us in our sicknesses and pains, even in our most appalling wretchedness, and we can find the way out of trouble.

If we tell Him what we suffer, what is on our hearts, and what comes into our minds, He takes it all and leads us in a process of healing with love and truth as we hear His responses, and as we check them with Scripture and accept them (for in this world there are many deceiving voices). This is affirmed in the Holy Bible, most particularly in Isaiah 53:4 and 1 Peter 2:24 and 3:10, and there are many present day Christians who will testify that it is true.

Be careful who you talk to about this sort of thing, however, because so many people still do not believe it - not even in churches - and many are bitterly opposed to it. Nevertheless, there are some folk who know and you will see the joy and peace in their eyes.

Jesus is coming back soon to reign in this world. The signs are there. Let us prepare to join Him (see Matthew 25:1-13 and Revelation 19:9). We shall each be called to account. He is Lord of all, and we do not want to fall into judgement. Let us allow Him to equip us for the place He has for us with Him in His kingdom.

By healing all our experience of this world, no matter what it may have been, He will build character within us that will eternally reflect His glory and be used in His kingdom to exercise His authority.

However much of a sinner you have been, whatever you have been through, however much you have suffered, however wretched you have been, be assured that are very precious to Him and that He has an eternal place for you.

THE FAITH

God is Spirit

If you get so desperate that you cry out "O my God!" or "God I can't take any more!" or "God! What is going on?" or "God! Help!" it seems you must be expecting there to be a god. So which god would you be calling to? To whom might you actually be appealing?

Is it a person? Is it a spiritual person you can't see? Can you really believe there is someone, some actual god, hearing you?

Let us be clear from the start about this sort of thing. There are many gods. Many spiritual beings would like you to believe that they are the only being that is almighty. There are many spirits who would like to be your one and only source of guidance. Each would like to have you for their own to mould you into their likeness, so that you will do their business.

If you find yourself in utter despair and then allow your mind and thoughts to become full of cursing and hopelessness, the spirit that comes upon you will be one that answers to your destructive state of mind. That spiritual being may seem quite nice and useful at first but it will prove to be deceptive and will eventually bring trouble upon you.

If any apparently useful answer to your desperation comes to mind you may at first feel better; but where will it lead? Will it lead to the helpful end you wanted when you first inadvertently called for spiritual help? Might some spiritual being actually demand your very life and end up destroying you?

Spiritual beings are powerful. Their influences give direction to people's thinking. They affect the mind profoundly. They take over people's lives. They empower people. They develop culture. They are used by persuasive people to manipulate others. - You could find you do not have the power, or even the willingness, simply to change your mind.

If you speak with someone with a different faith about personal matters, or about right and wrong, differences of opinion soon become obvious.

It is necessary, therefore, to be careful. In order to protect yourself, you'll need to be clear about which god you'll speak with. The only safe way is to use the name of the god you want. But addressing the god by name is not really enough. It proves to be essential to know the actual nature and person of that spiritual being, and to know whether or not you can trust and believe in that person.

Whoever you call on will come. If you get the wrong one you may live to regret it.

You will not usually see the spiritual being you call upon, and you may not feel any different. But after a while you may realize that your awareness and behavior and thinking have changed.

Good news

As the universe was created, and as life and love prevailed against death and destruction, usurping powers came into being, led by Satan. Human beings were seduced by Satan who empowered their minds to manage without God. But this brought deception and death. Human nature fell from perfection into sin. From then on we have had to fight against hardship and suffering, disease and madness in a world that tries to destroy us.

About four thousand years ago, however, in the land now named Iraq, Abram called out to the Creator of the universe. And Abram believed the replies he received. As a result, he left his home and travelled west. God the Creator changed Abram's name to 'Abraham', which means 'father of many'. And Abraham lived most of the rest of his life in the land now called Israel. And he prospered.

But Abraham had only one legitimate son, Isaac, and Isaac was astonishingly born when his parents were well beyond child-bearing age. Isaac continued the relationship that his father had had with God, and he too prospered. God found a wife for Isaac, named Rebecca. She bore him twins, named Esau and Jacob.

Only Jacob continued the same relationship with God. He, too, received a new name, 'Israel', and he, too, prospered. He had twelve sons, but some bad things happened. Joseph, next to the youngest, was sold as a slave into Egypt and eventually ended up in prison. Through exceptional circumstances, however, by interpreting a very significant dream, Joseph came into favour with the king of Egypt, Pharaoh. And, in consequence, Joseph was elevated to one of the highest positions in the country, and became responsible for preserving food supplies and distributing them during a prolonged famine. Joseph thus saved the lives of many people, including his own relatives. He found such favour with Pharaoh that his whole family was invited down into Egypt to live there.

The people of Israel prospered in Egypt through several generations and their numbers increased enormously. They lived closely together because they were farmers, whom the Egyptians considered to be too low a class of people to associate with. But when a new Pharaoh overcame the old dynasty of Egyptian kings the people of Israel were enslaved. Then life became very hard for them. The Egyptians felt threatened by the Israelites. They culled their numbers by killing their male babies. Moses, however, survived by a ruse whereby he was found before he died by Pharaoh's daughter. He was adopted by her so that he came to belong within the royal household. Eventually Moses led his people out of Egypt.

Extracting the people of Israel from Egypt involved overcoming and defeating all the spiritual powers that were controlling that nation. Moses had such a close relationship with the God of all creation that those gods of Egypt were supernaturally and systematically put out of action so that Israel could walk free. After they were liberated, Israel wandered in the desert for forty years. It took a long time for them to shake off their old Egyptian ways and to become strong enough to survive as an independent nation in the land we now call Israel. Although God repeatedly guided them and saved them, it was only to a limited extent that they became aware of Him. His ways and His ordinances nevertheless became part of their culture. They were a nation belonging to God, and they remain so to this day (see Romans 11).

Long ago, on their journey from Egypt, God revealed Himself to them as the God who heals (Exodus 15:26 and 23:25). So the Creator of the universe is the God of Abraham and of Israel. And He is the God who heals.

You can check all this with the Holy Bible.

Though the people of Israel have been rebellious, God has persisted with them for centuries. He provided leaders and prophets. When they did what was right with God, things went well and they prospered. When they failed to honour God or, worse still, when they worshipped other gods, things did not go well.

God's people Israel were even exiled from their land twice and scattered into other nations. Yet He has always had faithful people amongst them to this day.

Through His prophets He told them they would one day return to the land of Israel. Some returned from Babylon about two thousand five hundred years ago, but eventually they were exiled again. Yet in recent years many have returned for good, and they are continuing to do so, as was prophesied by Isaiah (Isaiah 11:11).

The patriarchs and prophets of Israel have handed down to us Holy Scriptures which have powerfully influenced civilizations throughout the world.

Exciting seductions of ways that were wrong with the Creator of the universe, however, have always seemed more likely to appease the immediate desires of the majority, including the people of Israel. We and they have worshipped many other gods and brought judgement upon ourselves by walking into the hands, and into the ways, of usurping spiritual beings whose purpose is ultimately to destroy. All of us have so often trampled God's love for us into the dust.

Yet God has never removed His hand from Israel. Though they are demonized by many, they remain His people to this day. In fact through them we see vital aspects of what God is doing in the world today. They are the apple (or pupil) of His eye (Zechariah 2:8).

Two thousand years ago God sent His only begotten Son to live amongst them. God loved this world so much that He became flesh and lived amongst the people of Israel in order to save all people from all over the world. We know this human Person as Messiah Jesus. In Hebrew He is called Yeshua HaMeshiach. He was born to a virgin called Miriam and lived in Nazareth, which is now a large town in Israel. As He grew up, He worked there as a carpenter with His father Joseph. When He was about thirty he became a travelling sage and took disciples. In those days Israel had a tradition of travelling sages. Jesus is reckoned by Jewish rabbis to be the greatest expounder of parables among them.

Whoever really met Jesus found in Him the power for absolute healing. Everyone who sought Him for healing was healed. He healed physical illnesses and drove out demons with a word. And people's minds, and their behaviour, were healed as people took Him into their hearts and accepted what he said. He taught that He would be present whenever people who truly know Him would genuinely gather into His name (Matthew 18:20). His healing is indeed found among us today.

The greatest thing Jesus did was to allow Himself to be arrested and condemned to death by the administrative authorities. They did not understand the full truth of what they were doing. They did not understand that He was God or that, being the only person who has ever been God-made-flesh, He is the only way to God. They did not understand that when they shed His blood He was actually paying the price to redeem the whole world from its fallen state. They did not understand that death could not hold Him and that He would rise from the dead and meet again with His disciples and eat with them before joining His Father in heaven. They did not understand that Satan and death and all the powers of this world would now be overcome. They did not understand that through His death and resurrection He demonstrated His victory over all other spiritual powers. Ultimate authority in heaven and in earth is His (Matthew 28:18). His victory is now for us to appropriate.

Jesus continues to intercede for us who live in this fallen world. To those who personally accept His redeeming sacrifice, God sends His Spirit. You do not have to be good. You only have to soften your heart and make it humble and forgive other people and repent. It is essential to recognize your sin and to be open about it with Him. He is entirely willing to forgive and redeem the very worst sinner.

Holy Spirit works in the lives of those who accept Him and who thank Him. He changes them. Their relationship with God is restored. They find themselves becoming equipped for the place He has for them with Him in His eternal kingdom. You can say this prayer to receive Him:

Almighty God,
Creator of the universe and God of Israel,
thank you for sending your only begotten Son, Messiah Jesus,
into this world to save sinners like me.
You know all things. And you know my heart.
I forgive those who have sinned against me, and I confess my own fallen nature and my sins.
I cannot manage without you.
I now accept that Jesus paid the price with His blood to redeem me.
Thank you, Jesus, for setting me free.
Thank you, almighty Father God, for saving me through Jesus and for bringing me into Your family.
Live in me by your Spirit.
Restore my life and equip me to be yours.
You are my God. I always want to be with you.
You will always be the One I worship.
I thank you and praise you and worship you.

THE TRUTH

No truth means no trust and no faith

Truth is the basis of security. Truth resonates with what is sound in our very being. You can trust what is true. You can believe those who speak truth. They inspire faith. Their authenticity encourages you to believe in them.

Even if truth sometimes makes facts hard to face, seeing in the light of truth reduces stress and invokes peace, because how it really is will not then be hidden, nor will it be unknown or threatening. The Bible tells that we are made in God's image; and truth is healing. Soundness in spirit, soul, mind and body comes from facing anxieties and painful issues in truth with God's help. We respond by being physically blessed when we can trust His presence even though we *"walk through the valley of the shadow of death"* (Psalm 23:4).

Truth is necessary in order to distinguish goodness from evil, and justice from corruption. And truth removes false guilt.

Untruth, falsehood, leads to misrepresentation, deception, discord, and confusion, which is a cause of mental illnesses - and of physical illnesses, too. When untruth is authoritatively declared to be true it undermines security, destabilises people and can eventually drive people crazy - either individually or collectively - causing terrible disturbance.

Many scientists declare proven facts to be the truth. Facts in themselves, and the uses to which they are put, however, do not have the powerful effect on people that truth has. We may not know all the relevant facts, and known facts may be selected to give a false picture. The significant relevance of facts can be misrepresented. Facts can be used for good or for evil.

Facts require interpretation. How they are used depends upon each person's thoughts, beliefs, desires and hopes.

Facts that seem relevant are taken into account in thinking, feeling and behaviour; but each person is motivated by unseen forces. Motivational thoughts often come out of the blue. Thoughts lead to actions. And all honest people will sometimes say, "I don't really know why I did that!"

The recognition that thoughts and feelings cannot always be trusted has made many people sceptical. Sceptics always retain some doubt. And with that little bit of doubt there will always be some hesitancy and anxiety about the authenticity and truth of their perceptions and motivations. This can never be totally remedied simply by consideration of all the facts.

Anyone seeking singleness of heart and action will actually be choosing to believe in, and to follow, an unseen higher power - a deity. They may not be fully aware of this; but whenever they make any appeal to intuition, or choose any idea for thinking and reasoning without humble and respectful reference to God, that is what will, in truth, be occurring. When they become aware that their perception and motivation seem to be helpfully guided, they will be beginning to trust a deity. That deity will be real. But there are many different deities. Each has a different personality. Each will claim to be true. Which of them can truly be trusted?

We shall know them by their ultimate fruits.

Jesus Christ proves to be the truth. To see all the facts through Him proves to be sound. It provides firm ground and brings peace (Jeremiah 32:39).

Truth is a person.

When Jesus says, *"Your eye is the lamp of your body"* (Luke 11:34), and when He says, *"If...the light within you is darkness, how great is that darkness"* (Matthew 6:23), He is speaking about perception. He is speaking about how clearly, how truthfully, we see.

Jesus says He is the light of the world. He says whoever follows Him shall not walk in darkness (John 8:12 KJV).

We follow Him by giving ourselves to Him with repentance and in trust, and allowing Him to live in us as Holy Spirit (John 17:23). This way, we find ourselves drawn to deny ourselves and to take up our cross and follow Him in opposition to lies, just as He did (Matthew 16:24). We find ourselves accepting wholeheartedly that Jesus' blood paid the price to redeem us all. We yield our lives to Him as our Lord every moment for His service and His glory, not loving our lives so much as to shrink from death (Revelation 12:11). Living this way we actually become more like Him and become agents for healing and peace in this world.

It is not a matter of trying. It is a matter of listening to Him and trusting.

It is not about believing that we should be doing this or that, nor is it about being stubborn, proud and headstrong and obeying a set of strict instructions and rules. Rather, it is simply about seeing what He is doing and following Him.

It is not about striving to be good. It is about allowing Him to check us, to reveal to us when we are not in accord with Him, and then allowing Him immediately to lead us in repentance and healing.

Jesus says His Spirit will guide us into all truth (John 16:13). This implies that our knowledge of His truth does not happen all at once, although it is always fully available to us. Although the people of God are in touch with the God of all power and truth and grace, therefore, Christians should never claim to have the monopoly on the truth of the moment. We are all fallible. We attend to what God is saying and doing, we listen to God's prophets and read Scripture, and if we are wise we know that God sometimes speaks through people who do not actually belong with Him. Jesus says His sheep know His voice and that His words never deviate from Scripture (John 10:4 and 35b, and John 17:17). We may trust the peace that comes from His Spirit when we perceive truthfully. But legalistic rules made by self-righteous Christians who think they know all the answers can lead to deception. *"'Not by might nor by power but by my Spirit,' says the Lord Almighty."* (Zechariah 4:6.)

As we receive His Holy Spirit to live in us, a process of sanctification begins. Once we begin to see things His way, He will build on it (Mark 4:24-25). The process of sanctification continues to mature us during the whole of our lives provided we do not stop it. As we get to know Him better, we find ourselves more in accord with Him and with His words in Scripture. As we disciple ourselves to Him, Jesus guides us and changes us to be closer to Him and more like Him. As we seek to heed Him in every aspect of our lives, sanctification heals the mind. This is the case even if it was really sick when we started.

Our ability to perceive His way improves with time. But to stay with Him we need courage to see and hear and understand His way in the face of a world that is perverse. Having our senses awakened by Him can be painful. For one thing, we discover new friends and new enemies.

Yet as He opens our eyes and ears and hearts to what is going on in this world and to what He is doing in it, He gives us courage. So we can really engage both with Him and also with the world. This way we actually find peace in the battle, and also healing for our minds.

His way is true (John 14:6). But our perceptions can often be faulty.

Assault on truth

God says His ways are not our ways (Isaiah 55:8). The ways of this world are not His ways. He asks us to adopt His ways (Matthew 6:10, Romans 12:2).

If we belong with Him, He will give us His discernment. It can be disturbing, however, to use His discernment in order to make true sense of all the words and meanings in everyday relationships, and of all the events that inevitably involve us. To find healing for the mind, however, it is necessary to see the world truthfully. And that can be distressing. But He will take the pain.

To stop it being painful by putting conflict and distress out of our minds, or by allowing it to confuse us, does not actually take the disturbance away. It only hides it.

Ephesians 5:11 says, *"Have nothing to do with the fruitless deeds of darkness, but rather expose them."* And Ephesians 5:14 says, *"…for it is light that makes everything visible. That is why it is said: "Wake up, O sleeper, rise from the dead, and Christ will shine on you.""*

People tend naturally to avoid truth that they find challenging. Seeing the truth of what is really going on can be too much for people who do not know Him. Then they get envious of those who see more clearly than they do. They do not like feeling challenged by stuff that exposes how it truly is. They prefer stuff that supports and confirms where they are at, stuff that entertains them with the compromises and messes they live with. Consequently they resist true healing and deny all possibility of it.

When Jesus returns to reign, faith will be stronger than it is now. There will be healing everywhere. But in the meantime people get envious of Christians and Jews who have a living relationship with the God of Israel, Creator of the universe. They hate the truth exposed by their very existence.

Healing the mind, and healing mental illness, therefore involves seeing through assumptions and concepts accepted by this world. It involves becoming a committed member of the family of Father God, rather than our own family. It involves belonging in the kingdom of God wherein Yeshua HaMeshiach, the Lord Jesus Christ, is both our king and our elder brother. Then we can take courage because He is with us. His Spirit living in us changes how we perceive, and heals our minds. If we tell Him our troubles and listen to Him he protects our hearts with His peace.

We should accept all the shrewdness He gives us. This world and its institutions, and all its various ways of thinking, will never really be sympathetic until Jesus comes back to change the world. We shall have enemies who seem to be friends. What appears to be kindness may actually hide cruelty. Therefore let those people who truly belong in God's family, those who know themselves redeemed by the very lifeblood of Jesus, pray for discernment and wisdom, trust in His guidance, and be polite and quiet but shrewd.

In practice it may well be necessary to live in conformity with many of the ways of the world, to respect its administrators, to pay taxes, to perform civic duties, to accept worldly qualifications, and so on, provided they do not compromise our integrity. It may be necessary, too, to use worldly academic, medical and scientific systems. We use them if we need to, but we do not put our faith in them. Our hope in God is our anchor (Hebrews 6:19).

We should expect spiritual attacks. Therefore we constantly keep His armour on, namely faith, truth, righteousness, salvation, the sword of the Spirit, shoes of readiness and constant prayer in the Spirit (Ephesians 6:13-18) and we stay alert in order to defend ourselves.

Essentially, attacks come only in two ways: from accusation and from deception. These are the only two weapons Satan has (as described in Revelation 12:9-11) but he uses them brilliantly.

Our armour and defence are essentially predicated upon our testimony that having accepted Jesus Christ, the only begotten Son of God, we are redeemed out of the hand of the devil by the shed blood of Jesus, the price He paid for us (Ephesians 1:7). When we truthfully make that declaration all our guilt and shame are gone, we cannot be destabilized, and Satan has no rights over us.

Satan knows whether or not he has any rights. And he knows the God of Israel has authority over him. The truth sets us free (John 8:32).

It follows that we need to make sure of being right with God. That involves allowing our relationship with God to change the way we perceive and think and behave so that we no longer conform to this world (Romans 12:2).

Certainly we shall all have been guilty of sin. Each one of us will have done wrong things and messed up, sometimes very badly indeed. Satan is quite capable of throwing up the memory of our wrongdoing into our consciousness. But when it has been brought into the light and confessed before God, thankfully accepting His forgiveness and the healing and the redemption that come from being washed with the blood of the Lord Jesus His Son (as in 1 John 1:7), the accusations of Satan are null and void, no matter how we feel. Then although accusations may be painful, they are ultimately unjust. So we can legitimately wear God's armour and use it to stand strong.

Deception is altogether more subtle. From people in authority saying one thing but meaning another (even parents, sometimes) to subliminal influences transmitted in music, deception is to be found everywhere. From influential people calling bad good and good bad, to sexual seduction; and from thrilling worship that is false, to pronouncements by religious leaders that are contrary to the word of God, deception pulls you into its tentacles. It can feel so good and seem so very much what you want, and so very reasonable. There is so much deception these days that we can say with Isaiah (59:14), *"truth has stumbled in the streets"*.

Everyone diagnosed with a neurotic or psychotic illness or a personality disorder will have yielded to the deceptions and accusations of the enemy in some way or other. Healing will always come, however, to anyone who comes with a humble heart and repentance to the Lord Jesus Christ and thankfully accepts His redeeming sacrifice, and who then diligently pursues a process of testing the spirits (1 John 4:1), facing the past, and allowing the blood of Jesus into the damage (1 John 1:7).

God desires truth in our inner being (Psalm 51:8 TLV). And there will be a reckoning.

THE MIND

Not an organ

The mental illnesses to which we are referring are not primarily illnesses that affect an organ. They cannot be sufficiently explained by anatomical or physiological pathology. They affect the mind. The mind is not an organ.

It is often unthinkingly assumed that the mind is in the brain. Because they reveal changes in the brain associated with mental activity, the disciplines of neuroimaging and neurophysiology tend to give that impression. And cleverly invented drugs are known to be used to sedate targeted sites in the brain in order to control behavior.

But there is no proof that what comes into the mind originates in the brain. Who knows where thoughts come from? If you are reminded of an idea, what you do with it comes from inspiration. If you ask God to show you something He may give an unexpectedly accurate answer. To assume that any particular organ is the seat of the mind must be wrong.

All we can truly say is that the mind is open to inspiration and connects with the sensory and motor activity of the body in the living state. We can also describe conditions of mind that affect perception and behaviour.

Listed here are some aspects of the activity of the mind. These aspects can act together at the same time in various combinations. This list simply expands the commonly accepted notion that the mind is about wanting, thinking and feeling.

Aspects of the mind

- There is discernment and perception. What is picked up by the senses is affected by spiritual influences, and ordered by reasoning with knowledge and imagination.

- There is awareness, anxiety, vigilance and warning. What is going on in the world, particularly in direct relation to the individual, arouses both assurances and anxieties in that person. Warnings serve to restrain behaviour. Too much anxiety clouds awareness.

- There is consciousness, whereby we are aware of what we are doing in relation both to our relationships in our external environment and to the extent of our inner peace.

- There is desire. Is this only instinctual? Are our desires only for air to breathe, for food and for love? It seems obvious that our desires are excited and directed by all sorts of relational, spiritual influences to which we allow ourselves to become attached, sometimes through seduction. To avoid being led all over the place, it would be better to be discussing all our longings with God.

- There is intention and will. Whether or not we know what we are doing, we direct our energies towards certain purposes. And we shall be held responsible both by the law of the land and also by almighty God, albeit according to rather different criteria. Our spirit drives us. Unless our human spirit is aligned with the Spirit of the Creator of the universe we shall ultimately have trouble.

- There is language and behaviour. Other people, other things, and all sorts of events affect us, and we respond. We seek understandings with other people.

- There is memory. What has been experienced and learned in the past affects how we think and behave in the present. Memory is called upon in order to make sense.

- There are habits and instincts. Inheritance plays a part, and genes are involved.

- There is emotion. It connects particularly with memories, and gives meaning to experience. Emotions are tempered by understanding and by empathy with others. The expression of emotion is spiritual. It will accord with the person's spiritual state, and with whoever is effectively being worshipped at the time. Those who know themselves to be redeemed and filled with Holy Spirit find they have the peace of God deep within their souls, with emotional stability and self-control (Galatians 5:23). Their emotional expression will accord with the will of God.

- There is reasoning, reckoning, understanding, conceptualization and belief, all of which is called 'cognition'. Many people really believe there is no need to refer to God. They believe what happens to come to mind after careful deduction will be good enough. They assume scientific, academic, legal and political deductions can be sufficiently sound. This way they may even believe mankind can save the world. When calamity hits, however, they will be proved wrong (see Matthew 7:24-27 and Matthew 24).

- There is concentration. We have an immense capacity to concentrate on a matter in hand, and to gather relevant considerations and use them creatively with inspiration and imagination.

- There is reflection, an ability to recollect with inspiration and receive spiritual guidance.

- There is recognition, an ability to use relevant knowledge, to empathize with other people, to know and to name from having known before.

- There is enjoyment with others.

- There is imagination, which is always driven by some desire or intention, which is creative, and influenced by relationships with other spiritual beings, including people.

- There is inspiration and revelation. We are profoundly influenced through our relationships. Spiritual influences come to us, directed by the person we effectively worship. Who do humanists or agnostics actually worship?

- Matters come to mind. In fact, we could say that the mind is constituted of what may come to mind. And if we are honest we must admit that we do not always know where a thought comes from, or why it has come. Some thoughts are obviously connected with the matter in hand. Other thoughts may have been put aside whilst we concentrate on the matter in hand, for example a person may put aside thoughts about which route to take whilst fixing the car for the journey. But then the thoughts about which route to take may intrude. Thoughts that are put aside like this, but which are readily available for consideration, are just under the surface, in the subconscious. But then there are other thoughts that come to mind out of the blue. Suddenly the person may find themselves thinking about car crashes. Now where would that come from? That sort of thing deserves further investigation. And it is often surprisingly useful, and potentially healing, to discover where this leads.

- There is peace of mind. Stress is reduced to minimum when we are hearing Holy Spirit like a voice behind us saying, *"This is the way; walk in it."* (Isaiah 30:21.) People who have accepted that God's only begotten Son, the Lord Jesus Christ, paid the price to redeem them from their fallen, sinful condition will receive Holy Spirit as they genuinely say, "Thank you." Holy Spirit will be working in their lives from then on, to change them and to heal them. But it is necessary to listen to Him, and to be shrewd in relation to the people of this world, even professional specialists, and even those closest to us. Healing comes by a process that takes time. And it is proof that we are indeed made in the image of God, who has created us to live with Him.

- There is a censor, too. The censor automatically cuts off conscious awareness of experiences or of thoughts that for the moment are irrelevant or too much. After the operation of the censor, stress and pain that could be overwhelming will be ignored. In very extreme instances this may even involve ignoring part of the body. Yet suppressed memory of intolerable experience will be stored away, and it may become the cause of later trouble.

- The way the mind works will affect the way the body functions. The way we act on our perceptions and thoughts inevitably affects the physiology and biochemistry of our bodies. Body language reflects a person's state of mind.

It is possible to think of other aspects of mind, too. In 2 Corinthians, for example, Paul speaks of imaginations, reasonings, speculations, arguments, knowledge and thought. The main point is that the mind is both sensitive to influences, which may be physical or spiritual or both, and also active and creative through connection with the physical body.

Heart and soul

We could also define the mind of a person as that aspect of the soul that may become conscious. We could describe the soul as the living principle of a person. The soul is constantly both physically and spiritually receptive and active, and influenced not only by what can be seen but also by what cannot be seen. Paul says, *"...what can be seen is temporary, but what cannot be seen is eternal"* (2 Corinthians 4:18).

So when we speak of the soul we are not describing an inanimate object. This personal soul is an individual presence confined within a living, physical body, and to be reckoned with in this world yet open to the eternal.

And when we speak of the heart, we are speaking here of the heart of the soul. It seems reasonable to assume that thoughts come together in the heart because the heart receives blood from every part of the living body. The Bible says, *"...the life of a creature is in the blood"* (Leviticus

17:11). And there is no good reason to suppose that this may not have an intimate bearing on the physical heart. After all, the physical heart does indeed respond to what we describe as the affairs of the heart, to what a person puts their desire, their will and their 'heart' into, and to those to whom the heart is given.

Thoughts of the heart are regulated by the brain.

Physiology, biochemistry, biophysics, genetics, and all such stuff studied by academic scientists, are aspects of the living physical body. And there is every reason to suppose that every aspect of the physical body is affected by the person's living mind.

We are unable totally to separate body, soul, heart, mind and spirit, because in a living person they all work together (but God sees below the surface, see Hebrews 4:12-13). The person must be considered as a totality.

Ultimately, what changes our present world, and what makes for health or disease, is who is worshipped. The Lord Jesus Christ is the Prince of peace (Isaiah 9:6).

At death, the physical body returns to the earth but the spirit and soul depart.

God knows the heart and knows those who are His

Judeo-Christian Scripture tells everyone to expect resurrection after death. We shall have a new eternal body. We are told that this will be followed by judgement, when we shall each be required to give a personal account before God. Those whose names are written in the Book of Life of the Son of God will be separated from those who go into permanent deadliness and torment.

There is no indication that God will accept excuses. There is no indication that He will accept mental illness as sufficient grounds for exoneration. He will expect each of us to have been responsible for all we have said and done (Matthew 12:33-37). So it seems best to get fit enough to keep short accounts with God by accepting freedom through Jesus, and not conforming to this world but being shrewd enough to find God's healing for the mind, and from so-called mental illness, no matter what this world's agents may say.

THE DAMAGE

Fallen world

Before we enquire into what may cause non-organic mental illness (broadly defined as neurosis, psychosis, and personality disorder) we must consider the damage done to human minds by our separation from God and fall from grace (Genesis 3).

It is commonly assumed that we are born with minds that have the potential to become healthy provided we have a careful upbringing and receive good education. But the world is full of set-backs. And from the moment we are born, if not from before, we survive against forces that could destroy us. And the responses of human beings, even the wisest of them, cannot be totally trusted.

Methods of education presume we can do as we are told; but we don't (see Romans 7). Although we intend to make good decisions based on available evidence, in practice we always fail to be totally guided by what we know to be right. The whole world is far from perfect. Although we think we can make everything all right, in practice we never do so. This world has fallen from grace, and our heredity affects us.

We shall not grasp the grace of God until we accept the redemption out of this fallen state provided by His only begotten Son the Lord Jesus Christ. Only when we come before Him in sincere personal repentance shall we begin to receive His Spirit which will guide us into soundness of mind, godly use of authority, and ease in loving and being loved (see 2 Timothy 1:7 KJV). This is in fact available for everyone (1 Timothy 4:10). It is the way to a healthy state of mind. But it involves battle against the fallen world we live in.

Administrative use of sedation

We must also decide whether the primary damage in mental illness is in the mind or in the physical system that regulates the mind, particularly the brain. The fact that drugs used as treatment for mental illness target sites in the brain seems to lead many people to assume that those drugs target the site of the illness.

But the mind is a function of the soul and no actual organ is found to be the seat of the mind. Therefore to target sites in an organ of the physical body with drugs must, logically, be inhibitory. Restricting the activity of a disordered person in this way will inevitably be experienced as oppressive. Such restriction cannot logically claim to be healing. Rather, it just checks and holds the person.

Holding the person with chemicals like this is usually done in order to limit nuisance, for the sake of other people, and occasionally for safety. And it may indeed sometimes give the person an opportunity to begin to find peace and healing.

Including God

Souls are individual, alive and immaterial. They are always involved with personal relationships. All personal relationships are essentially spiritual. Since the mind through its relationships is the executive part of the soul, it stands to reason that healing the damaged mind can only come about through relationships.

The mind changes according to who is believed. But advocates of all the different spiritual paths claim the potential for healing.

Those who are discerning, however, will see that every so-called god draws the person into commitment with effective worship, and eventually influences everything they do, and demands the total life of that person. Worship results in the person conforming more and more to the nature of the god who is worshipped. The purposes of that god will be worked out in their life.

The only god to offer both abundant life in this world and also eternal life in the next is the God of Abraham, Isaac and Israel whom Jesus Christ called Father. All other so-called gods lead ultimately to death. Any healing they offer proves bogus in the end.

Accusation and deception

Satan builds strongholds of control in people's minds using every conceivable tactic. His interest is in counterfeiting the word of God and in the death and destruction of human beings. He works through human beings and through demonic cultural influences. You can believe what really seems right, but it can turn out to have been contrived by mistaken influences ultimately deriving from the province of Satan. Yet he can disguise his activities to make them seem very attractive, reasonable and right. Not only that; but he often hides his tricks in plain sight. His methods can be summarized under two headings, namely accusation and deception, as related in Revelation 12:9-10.

Accusations hurt and wound. They come with shocks and abuse and terror and threats and hatred and rejection and slander and envy and extortion and deaths and all sorts of other serious nuisance. They make you feel guilty and they tempt you strongly to retaliate. Satan knows all your past mistakes, and your present weaknesses, and uses them and twists them with curses and mockery and arguments that may seem very reasonable. Curses and rejection can have particularly deadly effect. They can even make you ill. When they undermine your security, and seem justified according to the logic of this world, they dig deep into the soul. The only defence that works is to be active in thanksgiving, praise and worship, to live in accord with holy Scripture, to have dealt with all your sin in repentance before God, and to have accepted that Jesus has released you from curses, even inherited curses, by becoming a curse for you (Galatians 3:13-14). You forgive those who accuse and curse you, and you bless them (Luke 6:28). Then you will know yourself to be redeemed by the blood of Jesus, and you will be armed to stand strong against the enemy (1 Peter 2:6, Revelation 12:11).

Deception convinces you to believe what eventually turns out to be a lie. It works through unclean spirits that seem convincing, and through various forms of sorcery, and it wrecks your mind in a prolonged and subtle way. It inveigles your credibility with seduction and jealousy and manipulation and domination and intimidation, and so on. Eventually can cause perplexity, because something inside you gives you no peace, if you have succumbed to deception, for you were actually created to conform to the image of God (Genesis 1:27). The only remedy is to discover sound truth - the true facts and true relevance of past experience, and also the ability to discern truth in what is currently going on. Holy Spirit leads us into all truth, and through Holy Spirit, Scripture comes alive to reveal the nature of God, whose love and truth pose a challenge to us in this world.

- Discernment and perception can thus be distorted by camouflaging the pain of Satan's wounds. The complexity of his lies tempts premature closure, creating prejudices that control the mind.

- Awareness can similarly be blinkered, anxieties misconstrued. Vigilance and warnings become unnecessarily stressful. Prolonged worry, fear, guilt and shame can prevent a person being aware of the truth of much of what is going on.

- Consciousness can be limited to only what the person can bear, restricted by fears, prejudices and mental strongholds.

- Desires can be distorted by obsessive attachment to objects, ideas and people who falsely seem not only to be comforting and good, but also to be releasing. The path to real peace and godly fulfilment can be blocked by exciting addictions. Yet there is no real peace, and a deep inner frustration persists.

- Intention and will can be directed towards ends that are ultimately futile and harmful.

- Language and behaviour follow suit. They will reveal the extent to which restrictions of the mind imposed by the accusations and deceptions of the enemy cannot for the moment be overcome. But we shall each be accountable to God for every word we have spoken and for everything we have done. It is therefore best to persevere until it becomes possible to keep short accounts with God.

- Memories will be recalled to consciousness according to what appears relevant. But past distress can sometimes be too confusing, uncomfortable or frightening to recall; and therefore it may be ignored and left to fester. This can make a person ill.
- Habits and instincts will conform tenaciously to the restrictions imposed by the tricks of Satan. Every excuse under the sun will be used to avoid change.

- Self-control will be lacking for emotions not taken to the Lord for healing. Some expression of emotion may be so excessive or so offensive as to be socially sanctioned. In the parable of the sower, furthermore, Jesus speaks of worries and temptations that prevent the true understanding which bears good fruit (Matthew 13:1-23).

- Reasoning, conceptualization, cognition, and belief, will be influenced by unhealed wounds and deception - even when all the apparently relevant facts are considered. Wounds and deception twist thinking. We make up our minds under spiritual influences whether or not we are aware of them. Before you use your reason, therefore, it is necessary to decide whom you will worship.

- The ability to concentrate upon what is in hand can be interfered with by distractions as problems arise due to old wounds, and as uncertainties and misunderstandings develop due to faulty thinking.

- The ability to reflect, too, can be interfered with by the wounds of deceptive thinking.

- What is recognized and what is not may be determined by perception that is damaged.

- Enjoyment can not only lack inner peace but can develop into lustful frenzy under the hidden influences of satanic deception and unhealed wounds.

- Imagination can develop along damaging and ugly paths reflecting unhealed elements of the soul. This may actually seem advantageous, and may even pay well, because it can be used to create things that are fashionable. People like to feel they are amongst others with the same human failings. But the things of this world are ephemeral and one day we shall each be accountable to God.

- Inspiration and revelation are plainly under spiritual direction. Who wants them distorted by wounds of accusation and deception? Who wants tormenting voices?

- What happens to come to mind is determined not only by matters in hand and spiritual influences but also by unhealed wounds and distortions of thinking that prevent peace.

- Peace of mind is prevented by wounds of accusation and deception.

- Until there is healing, the censor will stop some issues coming to mind that need to be considered for truthful thinking.

- As distorted thinking leads to damaging behaviour, the physiology of the body will suffer. The finely tuned nervous and hormonal systems of the living body will inevitably be affected. This may make the body more susceptible to disease.

Hope

God told Isaiah to tell the people: *"You will be ever hearing, but never understanding; you will be ever seeing, but never perceiving. This people's heart has become calloused; they hardly hear with their ears, and they have closed their eyes. Otherwise they might see with their eyes, hear with their ears, understand with their hearts and turn and be healed."* (Isaiah 6:9-11, Septuagint.)

Those who truly accept Jesus as their savior, however, are given discernment to see and hear and understand. They will understand how the above distortions cause mental illness, and they will discover that Holy Spirit gives courage for changing their perception and thinking and healing the mind.

Sorting our minds out in truth may take a long time. It can be a painful process. But the Lord Jesus Christ of Nazareth will carry all the guilt and pain (Isaiah 53:4-6 and 1 Peter 2:24). Continuing to thank Him allows His healing grace and love to flood in and make us strong.

Those who persevere will discover that all serious mental illness has its origin in experiences of accusation, cursing, deception and abuse in early childhood before the age of about eight, before the age when a child has developed sufficient maturity to begin to make sense of the world. When the cause comes to light with the Lord, there is healing.

ANXIETY AND STRESS

Dire straits

Adverse conditions and perceived threats automatically cause us to be extra vigilant. We become ready for sudden emergency. We prepare for defence or escape, fight or flight, or both.

If the state of anticipation is at all prolonged we call it anxiety. Anxiety is an emotion that makes us physically and mentally tense, and ready for anything.

Bracing ourselves to meet the unknown causes stress, and stress uses extra energy. As we exert ourselves against adversity, even mild adversity, we use even more energy. Eventually the stress of constant anxiety and prolonged exertion can weary us and cause severe fatigue.

The response experienced as stress is mediated within the body by stress hormones. These are chemicals which cause our physiology to provide extra energy for immediate use. They also enhance our resistance to injury. But they reduce the sort of regenerative metabolism that takes place inside us when we are at peace, thereby reducing our long-term resilience. Scientists have discovered many of the anatomical, physiological, neurological and biochemical mechanisms.

Our alertness and preparedness will also involve emotional responses to our situation. Various stressful emotions will probably influence our reactions.

All emotion affects the body one way or another. Anticipatory and aggressive (fight or flight) emotions such as anxiety, fear, worry, anger, frustration, violence, produce physical stress. So does guilt. Peaceful, loving emotions, however, produce relaxation.

Stress can also be a result of trauma. Both the physical and the emotional effects of trauma produce severe stress.

If adverse conditions continue too long (for instance, during prolonged bombardment, or torture, or continual mental and emotional turmoil) stress uses up our reserves. Thus stress can eventually become seriously debilitating. Exhaustion can make us more likely to make dangerous mistakes in perception and in behaviour. Long term stress can make us more susceptible both to physical illness and mental breakdown.

There is a distinction between anxiety and stress which can be illustrated further:

If we are going to be interviewed for a new job we shall naturally be anxious, but the anxiety will soon pass. The stress will soon come to an end.

If we exercise very suddenly we shall be stressed, but we need not be anxious.

Concentrating on mental activity can also be stressful yet produce no anxiety.

Lack of sleep causes stress although it need not produce anxiety.

If we are anticipating a surgical operation, however, we shall inevitably be sufficiently anxious as to be somewhat stressed. During the operation the trauma will inevitably stress us, too. Recovery will take time. Continuing pain may cause anxiety and stress until there is healing. But the stress need not be grossly excessive.

If we are subjected to shock that has not been anticipated, anxiety only sets in after the event. Physical injury may also be involved. Stress will continue until both physical and emotional wounds are healed.

If we are frightened, and our frightening circumstances persist so long that there seems to be no option but to live with constant fear, the stress may eventually become seriously debilitating. If worrying circumstances persist we may become weary with anxiety and eventually feel ill. Both fear and worry are often simply called anxiety.

If we are persistently frustrated and angry we shall be stressed with all the emotion, although we may not feel particularly anxious. If we carry a load of guilt that we have not confessed to God, and for which we have not accepted the forgiveness provided by Jesus, we shall carry the stress of it, whether we are aware of it or not. If we find no healing for our emotional state, our deeply unsettled reactions are likely to produce circumstances that worry us. Anxieties and worries will then be added to our emotional burden.

Prolonged emotional tension that becomes a chronic state of mind will cause chronically debilitating stress that may predispose or contribute to mental or physical sickness.

Hidden conflicts

Thus anxiety and stress may come from outside us or from inside us. The anxiety and stress inside us come from experiences during our lifetime that have not been healed.

In childhood we are usually protected by our parents. They put our experiences and perceptions into context by explaining them and reassuring us. Yet that is not always the case. From the very beginning of some people's lives there may have been experiences which they have never been able to make sense of. If there is too much of that sort of trauma, the child cannot concentrate on anything. This causes **Attention Deficit Disorder, 'ADD'**. For a surprising number of people some experiences may have been overwhelmingly confusing, distressing or frightening. Rejection, abuse, loss and grief are common. The distress will be remembered; but the memory may be confusing. And it is often never brought to light or discussed; it is rather suppressed, and covered over by putting on a good face. This causes constant, hidden stress, and some people live with it all the time.

Peer group pressure, and addiction to social media, may make it easy to avoid uncomfortable memories and thoughts that should be opened up and healed.

Inherited tendencies influence a person deeply causing prejudices and ways of thinking that obscure truth. Many profound spiritual influences from the cultures our ancestors have lived in, and also from the culture we currently live in, are subtly stressful and seldom fully understood.

Inherited curses, too, can blight one's life with hidden stress. So can hidden guilt.

With maturity there comes greater understanding. Sometimes it will be possible to come to terms fairly easily with distressing events and with harmful influences that have caused difficulties in the past. But there are many mature people who have never been able to make sense of childhood events, and who remain chronically troubled in consequence without really knowing why.

Furthermore there are many people who have been confused or traumatised so severely as adults that they have never been able even to think about it. This is the stuff of nightmares. Experiences from wartime and experiences of accidents or torture are notorious.

Experiences and perceptions that are too much to handle are frequently censored automatically by the human mind. They are put out of mind. The memory, however, remains buried in the soul, in the 'unconscious', too threatening ever to recall. Nevertheless it remains a hidden influence. Whenever recall happens to be threatened by a reminder, a trigger immediately says, "Don't go there!" Many people have serious hang-ups of this sort.

So we may find ourselves living with anxieties we cannot understand, in a chronically stressed state, perhaps even a depressed or crazy state, due to unconscious material that we are not aware of.

The effects of long term stress can eventually be exhausting and shattering. It can actually be the cause of chronic hypersensitivities and allergies, susceptibility to infections, weakness, endocrine disorders, arthritis, rheumatism, and severe, chronic psychiatric illness.

We only discover the cause, and find the healing, when a time and place arrives that is safe and conducive enough for the light of truth to be shed upon distressing events.

Such a facilitating environment can sometimes be found through meeting in a very open way with other people who have had similar experiences. Speaking together about past distressing events with other people who know what you are talking about, and who are attempting together to gain greater understanding and healing, can be liberating. We commonly find surprising empathy, compassion and comfort amongst fellow sufferers. It needs to be safe, however, for every participant to become vulnerable. Such meetings should therefore be refereed by people of integrity and deep understanding, in order to prevent exploitation of vulnerable individuals and abuse of their weaknesses and revelations. And of course it is best if everyone involved will bring their distresses and vulnerabilities to the Lord.

This sort of group therapy was used in a secular way in the past in the psychiatric services, in the armed services and in prisons, and considerable healing was achieved.

As many different faiths have become predominant among us now, however, it proves to be surprisingly difficult to persuade secular politicians, administrators and actuaries to facilitate and fund this sort of group therapy, probably because of a perceived potential for litigation, since different mores and standards can cause offence to different faiths. In a secular, multi-faith society, responsibility for one's actions can only be assumed if distinct illnesses are scientifically categorised, so that sufferers can be diagnosed and treated, rather than spiritually challenged and assisted, when self-control fails. Secular treatment of the mind must therefore be seen to be done with drugs and scientific psychological manipulation, which are easily quantifiable, and therefore explainable and acceptable as an expense.

Outside of a Judeo-Christian culture there is deep-seated resistance to the terrifying idea that letting down one's defences in humility, and understanding them, could ever eventually result in peace of mind.

Hidden conflicts can thus be seen to reside not only in the unconscious minds of individuals but also in society as a whole and in government. In consequence, those with mental distress in a secular society tend never to be truly understood, always consequently frustrated, always considered insane, and relegated to a place beyond the pale, outside the city gate. This way, shame attaches to mental illness. And the diagnosis and the stigma become a curse.

A secular institution will therefore never be a safe place for all this to be undone and overcome. Healing must be found amongst the genuine people of God.

Peace

It helps to have the encouragement of others who really know the Lord. They need to be patient with us in our pilgrimage, hospitable, ready to listen, with enough self-discipline to avoid offering good advice with premature judgement. The empathy, understanding, prayer and support of Christians not conformed to the world is important. Galatians 6:2 & 5 encourage us to carry one another's burdens in such a way as to enable each to carry his or her own load. Off-loading stress and anxiety onto the cross, discerning between truth and deception, and changing the mind about all sorts of issues, is a process that takes time.

God is merciful to those who fear Him, who honour Him with thanks and praise and worship, and who maintain their relationship with Him, and hear His words. His Spirit will continue to reveal the facts of our lives, past and present, in the light of His truth, until we really receive His healing and peace. If we stay willing to repent, and build trust in Him, and constantly get to know Him through Scripture, we shall tend to keep right with Him so that His truth will set us free (John 8:31-32).

At specific moments and places which He will provide for our personal healing, He will reveal matters that have been put out of mind. It will be safe, then, to face them with Him. He will show us the way out of dilemmas.

It often helps to have a specific person you can trust with whom to speak, to open things out with, who will not get in the way of what God is doing.

The process is often a battle. It is necessary to persevere and endure and never give up. It is necessary to remember that He enables us to forgive, and He forgives us when we repent. When we accept the sacrifice Jesus made for us, He removes our guilt.

It is necessary to remember that authority over all the power of the enemy is given to disciples of Jesus (Matthew 10:1) and that disciples do not have to be perfect before they are delivered from unclean spirits. They only have to use the authority given to them to resist the enemy and expel him from their souls - usually through their breath with a cough or a vomit.

"God is our refuge and strength, an ever-present help in trouble." (Psalm 46:1.)

God heals the wounds of all who come to Him in the name of Jesus. He changes the way we think and gives us new life. This is a process of sanctification, of becoming increasingly at peace with God, and it heals mental illness.

CHRONIC FATIGUE (M.E.)

When long-lasting emotional stress is suddenly bombarded with an acute physical stress which more or less puts you to bed, perhaps due to a severe viral illness like influenza, tiredness and weakness can sometimes persist, with muscle and joint pains, for a long time afterwards until eventually your strength returns. Such a condition sometimes goes under the name of M.E., or myalgic encephalomyelitis, signifying chronic, painful weariness of body and mind, and lack of resilience which proves difficult to overcome. It makes a person want to lie around all day and do nothing, longing for greater rest.

Both physical and spiritual components may be recognized. Both mental and muscle fatigue can be seen to be a physiological result of chronic stress of an emotional, spiritual and physical nature. The particular neuron connections to muscle that control muscle tension may be damaged by a virus, or perhaps by depletion of essential nutrients (as also found, for example, in the rare disease of scurvy).

It is necessary to discover before God what the original, long-standing stress was, which rendered the acute stress so debilitating. If you ask the Lord, He will show you. You will need to look inside your own soul and ask the Lord to assist your repentance.

It is often, but not always, the case in this condition that the pattern of current, close interpersonal relationships is similar to the pattern of relationships in one's childhood family. So then the pattern of current relationships is familiar - so familiar, in fact, that relationships and attitudes which were wrong with God, such as unrighteous issues and unfinished business that could never be put right in one's original family, are carried over habitually and unthinkingly into present relationships. This may turn out to have been the cause of the long-standing stress you were scarcely aware of until you got the flu.

Of course there are other reasons for chronic stress, such as onerous duty. Hatred and cursing from other people can wear you out, too. Or the culture surrounding you may be spiritually poisonous.

If you are open to all these sorts of possibility, and willing to be brutally honest with yourself, issues that the Lord brings to mind can be dealt with before God in the name of Jesus. You will need to give your pain and stress to the Lord Jesus, and thank Him for taking it from you at the cross (Isaiah 53:4). You can be forgiven for your mistakes. Those who have sinned against you can be forgiven. Unclean spirits can be expelled. God will heal both your impoverished spirit and also your body. He will also heal your current relationships; although it would be a mistake to expect those around you to change.

It may be necessary to take time out, with rest and a good diet, in order to come to terms with the condition you are in and to seek the Lord.

Sabbath rest

"There remains, then, a Sabbath-rest for the people of God; for anyone who enters God's rest also rests from his own work, just as God did from His. Let us, therefore, make every effort to enter that rest, so that no-one will fall..." (Hebrews 4:9-11).

24 hours of rest every 7 days are necessary for the health of most working people. A weekly Sabbath can be a special time for sorting out the heart and mind and aligning oneself with the mind of God. (This is not a recommendation for being religious at church once a week, but for rather personally resting in the Lord.) Healing time like this helps us persevere, even when we are in relative health, and enables us to keep His rest and peace in our hearts all the time whatever our circumstances.

DEPRESSION

Depression need not be an illness

Quite naturally there are times when it is entirely appropriate to be miserable. Set-backs are common. Misunderstandings can be deeply distressing. We make terrible mistakes. Accidents occur. Shocks shake us up. There are disappointments, failures and deaths. Loss can be dreadful. Illness may linger. Confusion and pain may be prolonged. Information overload deadens the mind. Other people wound us. Enemies may abound. Rejection is painful. 'Black Dog' may be inherited. Oppression can be political. Constant stress may deplete the energy needed to prevail.

Substance abuse is very common and often becomes addictive. Addiction can make us depressed particularly by producing profound regrets. Addictions sometimes cause appalling things to happen.

Reminders of deaths, disasters and tragedies that have occurred in adult life can make people desperate enough totally to suppress any thought of what happened. Prisoners of war exposed to horrendous torture and deprivation will never go there again because the emotions and thoughts aroused are too disturbing.

Full recall can be too much for an individual to cope with, too stressful physically and constantly too mentally tormenting. Sometimes it seems that any suggestion that could lead to fully remembering could quickly lead to emotional overload, rage, weeping, and hopelessness, even a sense of worthlessness and a desire for death.

Hidden conflict and confusion, hatred, unwillingness to forgive, rage, sadness, self-pity, resentment, etc., often play a big part.

But unfinished business deep in the soul may always be brought to light and dealt with at the cross of Jesus. He never gives us more than we can cope with at a time (1Corinthians 10:13). And He knows it all, He has been there, and He has in fact overcome it. We may appropriate the healing He provides by beginning to tell Him about it. If we accept His presence, that very acceptance allows Him into our lives and He will begin to affect us and change us.

Those joyful people seen on Christian websites give an impression that to be Christian you have to be carefree. They persuade you to believe it necessary always to be smiling and happy if you belong to any Christian church. Frankly, there is some uncomfortable truth in that these days. Many Christians get so passionate about praise and worship that they avoid the reality of suffering. They think you should always put on a positive face that other people will 'like'. They may even dismiss you with condescending words if you reveal how you really feel. It can be necessary to come out from being amongst those sorts of Christians.

Because distress and wretchedness are not well tolerated or understood, misery has become medicalized. We go to the doctor with it. Most doctors, will treat it with drugs or with psychological techniques because they, too, find it too painful to tolerate, and too time-consuming to empathize with. After all, medicine must be scientific and secular these days. There is little time, or wisdom, for healing relationships, and no room for spiritual considerations. Unless the true causes are faced, however, rather than only the biochemical and physiological concomitants, we shall live in some degree of unreality. And our security, both personal and collective, will diminish in consequence.

Suffering is allowing the reality of how hard it is to work through all our human failings and mess. Unless an individual personally makes time and space available with God for working through what must be suffered, there will eventually only be pain. Pain can be overcome, however, by addressing the real issues with God.

If such issues are not tackled, the pain of distress and wretchedness can cause despair to get worse. Despondency and hopelessness follow. Worthlessness and rejection set in. Self-pity and resentment increase. It becomes harder and harder to forgive those who have wronged you, and to seek forgiveness and healing.

Medication

Medication will often kill the pain, ease the stress and lift the mood. Antidepressants can keep a person functioning at work. An antidepressant drug may seem like a wonderful cure. But it will anaesthetize the person against the full import of reality, and may hinder real healing. Youngsters with no time for suffering, however, often seek no other remedy.

There is a proper place for medication, of course. It can hold you, if all seems lost.

But antidepressants make big profits for the pharmaceutical industry. And the vast number of people taking antidepressants can be seen as an indication of a lack of trust in anything but drugs and human ingenuity for the relief of human wretchedness - and also as an indictment upon Christian congregations.

Drugs alter perception and behaviour. The use of drugs that affect the mind is a form of sorcery for manipulating us.

If time and space can be made for addressing the real issues, antidepressant drugs are often not needed at all. After all, high quality time and space can be found privately with God behind a closed door.

Patience

Many people who break down, however, cannot figure out enough of the reason why they should feel so bad. They really cannot say why they are depressed, nor can they speak about it much at all. Lack of energy, lack of sleep, lack of interest, a sense of hopelessness and frustration, self-neglect and torment, just seem overwhelming.

It may help to have another human being, or a professional psychotherapist, with whom to explore the sense of what may have been going on. But it can be hard these days to find anyone with wisdom who truly understands.

It may be wisest to begin to try privately to describe for yourself how you are feeling. There are hidden influences in the mind that can be explored productively by waiting on God. Informative connections can be made. The discipline of regularly making time and space to rest, and simply to allow matters to come up into the mind without censorship, is of enormous benefit. If you persist in telling God about it, and if you let Jesus His Son take any conflict and pain (Isaiah 53:4), and listen for His guidance, peace will eventually come. Painting, writing, or music making, or some other sort of simple creativity, may help some people to begin to do this.

Depression can be like a room inside you; and rooms have doors: the way in is the way out. It is wise to get into the truth of what has been going on and how you feel and think, even though it may be uncomfortable. There is no need to be self-critical about being self-absorbed, for there is very necessary private work to be done with God, and healing is definitely available.

Full insight is not always a prerequisite for a fair measure of healing. Sometimes people just need time and space to catch up with themselves, time for reflection, or sufficient 'drifting' time like the time between sleeping and waking. Things come to mind during such dreamy times, and connections are often made that become healing. Connections build sense and, when true sense eventually becomes apparent, there is relief. So with sufficient rest, and by the grace of God, a sense of healing may come, often with some degree of insight and understanding.

If we turn to the Bible we find many people whose wretchedness is recorded. Jacob, Joseph, Job and Moses, Elijah, David and Hosea, Jeremiah, Ezekiel and Daniel, and Jesus Himself, and Paul, all went through times of very considerable despair and suffering. The book of Hebrews tells us Jesus was made perfect, and learned obedience, through suffering (Hebrews 2:10-11 and 5:8) and it gives a list in 11:32-38 of those "*whose weakness was turned to strength*".

In Proverbs 17:3 it says, "*The crucible for silver and the furnace for gold, but the Lord tests the heart.*" In depression God is testing us. So let us be reassured by Deuteronomy 4:7 where the word of God says, "*...the Lord our God is near us whenever we pray to Him.*" This is the case even when we are not aware of His presence. The ongoing use of prayer, opening the heart privately to the Lord (see Psalm 62:8), and frequent use of the Bible, may be all that is necessary.

If the misery is allowed to take its course with God's wise guidance, and if harmful interference is avoided, there will eventually be found to have been something brewing inside the soul. In due course it will be found that some changes have been made. It may even be as if the depression has been like a sort of pregnancy, and its resolution a sort of new birth.

Attack

There is an enemy that wants people dead (1 Peter 5:8). And there is a loving Father who wants us to live with Him. The Father has a job for each one of us, and depression may be part of the trouble that it is necessary to go through in order to get fit and become equipped (Psalm 119:71). The enemy will certainly do all he can to interfere with such a process and stop it. Thus there is a constant spiritual war. Each one of us should be fully aware of this war. It is a matter of survival. The forces of death are all around us. We fight them with Holy Spirit.

Eternal life is available to all who accept a personal relationship with the Lord Jesus, the only begotten Son of God, who gave His life to save everyone, and rose from the dead. Those who accept Him belong in His Father's eternal family. It is not only a family, however, but also a kingdom, composed of those for whom the Lord Jesus is king with eternal authority. And it is also an army that fights a good fight in this world (1 Timothy 6:12) with weapons that have *"divine power to demolish strongholds"* (2 Corinthians 10:4-5). The God of Israel will equip us for battle and give us His armour (Ephesians 6:14-18). Victory comes through listening to Him.

It is necessary to be aware of the enemy's tactics.

One way or another, the accuser will throw at you everything you ever did that appears wrong. And he treats you very badly through other people. We need both to forgive all others who have offended us and also to know ourselves not guilty, forgiven and healed.

To avoid deception it is essential to note most carefully that what God says will never deviate from Holy Scripture.

First of all it is necessary to discern truth. After you have genuinely accepted Jesus Christ you will discover that you no longer perceive as the rest of the world perceives. Although you may be tempted to conform to the society you have always kept, there will be a quietly persistent voice within you showing you a different way that accords with the truth of almighty God. Old friends may fall away and new friends appear. You may also discover that some of the opinions and judgements of parents and teachers and professionals are actually wrong (Luke 14:26 and 18:29-30). If this should be so, the Lord will show you what to do about it.

There is usually no point in agitating for social justice because that belongs to the politics of the fallen world we live in. It is necessary to remember that the secular world does not believe in God and does not believe He heals. This world will only change when Jesus returns. We only need to be allowed to let our light shine (Matthew 5:16).

If you are suffering from depression, it is probable that the opinions and judgements and deceptions and accusations of other people throughout your life will have worn off on you. And most probably you will have responded according to your fallen human nature. You may naturally be bitter, angry, full of resentment and self-pity, defeated and sullen, fearful and guarded. Many of those responses will have become habitual, so that when circumstances arise that are similar to circumstances that caused those bad reactions in the first place your responses will be similar.

Sometimes the rage, or other emotion, from an earlier offence against you may be acted out much later. I remember a man who had been sexually assaulted by some girls when he was a young boy eventually being sent to prison as a grown man for rape. Old wounds that you thought were buried may raise their ugly heads until they are healed.

Desperate situations that have produced desperate responses may have let unclean spirits in. If unclean spirits are there, the Spirit of truth (John 14:17) will reveal them. They will manifest themselves. If so, it is necessary to repent before the Lord and to forgive all people who have wronged us. We may then receive God's forgiveness and healing by accepting that Jesus' blood was shed to pay the price to redeem us. If we accept this, we can then command each unclean spirit to go in Jesus' name. We expel them with the authority He has given us (as in Matthew 10:1 and Revelation 12:11). Demons often come out with a cough or vomit.

Healing the mind takes time, sometimes a long time, usually a lifetime. It is a matter of discerning truth, of repentance and forgiveness, and of getting rid of unclean spirits. It can be a mistake to expect immediate relief. Like good wine, we mature in God's timing.

Post-natal depression

It is astonishing to realise how many women there are whose post-natal depression seems connected with bad experiences during childbirth. Lack of empathetic understanding and compassion in the increasingly defensive practice of scientific obstetrics has wounded many women when they have been particularly vulnerable. A willingness to forgive their medical attendants or other influential people is essential for their own healing, no matter whether forgiveness is deserved or not. They may themselves need God's forgiveness, too, for having had unrealistic expectations of scientific medicine.

Of course, there may be other factors carried by the mother that have predisposed her to be sad and wretched after the birth, such as worry, fear, bitterness, hatred, rejection, and so on. But as she tells God about it all, and thankfully accepts the victory of Jesus over all the trouble and pain, she will find healing. As she receives comfort from Holy Spirit, He will enhance the love she shares with her child. And He will open the way for her to cope.

OBSESSION

Obsessive Compulsive Disorder

Should it ever happen that a young child below the age of about eight is actually seduced into sexual activity, that child would be too young to understand the full import. The sexual activity would most likely be initiated by an adult. Therefore the experience would prove to be beyond the capacity of the child fully to comprehend. Probably it would be confusing and frightening, and possibly eventually overwhelming as more of the implications became apparent. Even if the sexual activity were initiated by another child, there would have been some connection with an adult at some stage, and the nature of the activity would be adult, and consequently beyond the capacity of the child to take full account of. Confusion and fear might be exacerbated by the aggression, guilt, shame and disgust of the perpetrator. To destroy the evidence, children have sometimes actually been murdered. If the child survives, the child will live with the not-fully- realised memories, the confusion, the fear, hidden guilt, and also, possibly, the consequent sexual precocity. If there were no terrifying threats, the child could become accustomed to secret sexual activity and only realise later the shameful and socially unacceptable nature of what occurred. Secrecy will be demanded. All the memories and emotions will therefore be repressed, and the child will learn to behave as if none of it ever happened.

The innate desire of the child's soul for ease and peace will, however, have been thwarted. The child is likely to grow up with hidden fear, confusion, shame and guilt and excessive sexual desires. But all this will have been repressed and buried in the unconscious order to keep the secrets secret. The child will have developed an ability to put on a good face, so as to fit in within the family and the school and the workplace and amongst friends and acquaintances. Hidden pressures, however, will guide the mind to be diverted from anything that could allow really conflicting buried secret issues to come into full conscious awareness. Yet there may be excessive seductiveness or excessive masturbation. And a pervasive interest in sex, and also an attraction to people and circumstances similar to those originally involved, may initiate various adventures, some of which may also be remembered as disturbing, and some of which may be dangerous. The true nature, and the full facts about the original causes, of the hidden stress the person lives with will, however, be kept firmly out of mind.

If any event or activity of the mind really threatens to remind the person powerfully of the original secret details, activity will immediately be displaced and diverted into something inconsequential.

In this way a compulsive habit can develop, like compulsive handwashing, for example. It will be used to keep forbidden secrets hidden, although the individual may not be aware that this is actually the case. And a fearful, stressful urgency, essential for maintaining a good-enough face, and for maintaining secrecy, and for avoiding mental breakdown, will make certain the compulsive habit will never be relinquished by human effort.

Sexual abuse in childhood is not the only cause of pathological obsessions, however. Other unspeakable events (such as illegal cruelty, or threats) may certainly be implicated.

Driven by powerful emotions connected with issues of which the person is not actually conscious, the compulsive habit may be concentrated upon some object, idea, fantasy or person - anything that effectively diverts the mind. If the temptation to indulge the habit is resisted (and the compulsion is often hated) the temptation to do it becomes stronger. Thus anxiety and stress will increase, and with it self-justification. A fear develops that failure to appease the compulsion will induce calamity. So excitement and stress increase. Then yielding to the compulsion brings relief.

The person is effectively enslaved.

The majority of compulsive acts are concerned with cleaning (like hand-washing). The majority of obsessive thoughts, which may occur instead, are to do with checking. Persistent ruminations combined with impulses to act may, however, be about all manner of things, from a compulsion to change sex, to a compulsion suddenly to expose the genitals, to feeling compelled to touch a certain object, or an obsession with a certain person. Obsessions and compulsions can become very distressing. They can make a person feel desperately hopeless and depressed.

Tics

Twisting the body suddenly, in some repetitive way, or calling out suddenly maybe with obscenity (as in Gilles de la Tourette syndrome), are called tics. Their origin is similar. They usually seem to be triggered by some subtle thought directly or indirectly connected with childhood trauma, or by a reminder of unfinished childhood business, that the person is not actually conscious of. Their origin is similar to other compulsions. They are a cover for something that has never come to light. But God will reveal it in His good timing if He is invited to do so in Jesus' name. Then there can be healing.

Displacement

Powerful emotional responses of the soul are entirely natural in the face of turmoil or abuse of the person. They are often exaggerated after the event by concocted imaginings and dreams, especially if the person has not understood the full import of what occurred. If the turmoil or abuse occurred before the age of about eight, the memory will be repressed into the unconscious. If such natural responses have occurred in a more mature individual, and if they are powerfully frustrated due to perceived social sanctions, they will be suppressed; but memories of the turmoil or abuse will remain hidden and continue to fester, accompanied by subsequent imaginative elaborations and fantasies. Consequently the urge for expression may be diverted elsewhere and displaced for relief. Temptation comes along. The urges and desires of the soul may be displaced onto another object, idea, activity or person that seems to offer some alleviation. Relief will then be felt; but it will be exaggerated, because all the stresses involved in the build-up will, for the moment, be dispersed. This build-up followed by relief is found in all addictions.

Whatever the full truth may be about a person's obsessions or addictions, God knows all the details (Hebrews 4:13) and He desires that people turn to Him for peace and healing. The fullest relief comes from bringing the full truth to light and dealing with it in the light of Jesus. This is usually a process that takes time.

Phobia

Some people become obsessed with fear. Irrational fears hiding uncomfortable unconscious memories plague the lives of multitudes of people. Fears of mice or spiders, fears of contamination and pollution, fears of eating certain foods, fear of flying, fear of sexual feelings, fear of going out, fear of crowds, fear of heights - all these are common. And they provide material for superstition.

The objects feared are not actually the basic problem. The basic problem is the origin of the fear. And only with patience and perseverance will it become evident that the fear has been displaced in the course of time from an original confusing terror, usually experienced in childhood, and put onto certain objects, situations, ideas, activities or people.

Really sustained anxieties and chronic fears may even cause such chronic stresses that the person becomes exhausted without realising why. In such a case, the immune system becomes over-taxed. So does the mind. And mind or body may react with abnormally acute shock at even the slightest unaccustomed event. Then some actual substance that seems odd or strange may become the cause of allergic reaction. The body will have become so depleted of reserves that it can no longer defend itself with full immunity. Asthma, hay-fever, eczema, food allergy, and even some cases of diarrhoea and fainting, can thus be the result of a persistent spirit of fear, from which the person can be delivered in the name of the Lord Jesus.

In this context it must also be mentioned that the suffix '-phobia' has been misused and attached for political reasons to various words such as 'homosexuality' or 'Islam' or other contentious subjects. There has clearly been an intention to manipulate people into fear of expressing criticism. This is a misuse of the meaning of 'phobia', for it is logically untenable. Even the most prejudiced person cannot be accused of irrational fear or phobia unless fear actually exists in the person. Perceived prejudice, furthermore, need not be irrational. It may represent no more than a conflict between different systems of belief, and different deities.

Addiction

Some people become obsessed with substances that relieve stress. You can get some of those substances on prescription. Sleeping pills and sedatives are horrendously addictive. Anything to kill the pain - heroin, cocaine, tobacco, alcohol - all provide a 'feel-good' semblance of comfort. Music can be used to blank out the mind, too. So can social media. Video games and films give vicarious outlet to emotional reactions that seem to have nowhere to go. Some folk become obsessed with impersonal sex, pornography, prostitution. Some even become addicted to ice cream - anything for a little comfort in order to keep going. It can seem these days that there is no time to dwell on trouble, loneliness, meaninglessness, isolation and pain. Many believe any search for true compassion, empathy, understanding or love to be pointless. But that is a cop-out and a lie.

For some desperate people pain can be the only thing that seems real. Adrenaline junkies, and addicted gamblers, are so lost that the only thing they enjoy is the battle to get the substance or fix and the next high.

Many Christians have failed to connect the word of God in the Bible with the actual nitty-gritty of everyday struggle. The poor in spirit have been neglected. There has been a failure to connect the gospel of Jesus Christ with the wretchedness of the fallen world. We so easily forget that Jesus himself loves sinners and was made perfect through suffering (Hebrews 2:10 and 5:8-9).

The health service provides drugs to keep people at work. The government tries to tell you how to think. Universities leave no room for any sort of critical thinking which could possibly be so distressing as to interfere with a successful career. There is no room for people to be upset. Everyone seems to have an urgent need to concentrate on achieving sufficient success in order to keep going and survive. Everything must seem all right and be controlled by the state for us to be productive.

Theologians have been too worried about their academic jobs to allow themselves to be aware of what is really going on. Mental struggle and suffering are to be suppressed by psychiatrists. Let us all just love one another! We want no more pain, no more war. Let the government control everything, including our money, our families and our jobs. Opium for the masses – feed them with drugs. We live in a drug culture. Reality is lost. Truth is lost. No wonder so many people are addicted. What else are we free to believe in? Everyone is addicted to self-effort for survival. Antichrist is coming.

Frustration with unreality, with all the associated issues, needs particular attention.

Receiving the only begotten Son of the Creator of the universe, Messiah Jesus, as your Lord and Saviour redeems you from all that. Thanking the Lord Jesus for what he suffered for you on the cross, and speaking out your thanks, is the beginning of receiving Holy Spirit. When He lives in you, you'll see things differently. When you suffer you'll remain on a firm foundation. Jesus will take the pain. Tell Him about it. He holds you. You will find the Lord Jesus understands and brings peace. Your wounds heal. Slavery to substances, and to manipulation, and to your unconscious, is overcome. You move on. You stop stressing. It is not the sort of peace the world gives (John 14:27 and 16:33). It is an eternal peace that encourages and strengthens you and provides a new lease of life with the Prince of peace Himself. Self-control just happens, as a by-product (Galatians 5:22-23).

Anorexia

Like many other medical labels, 'anorexia nervosa' is simply a description in Latin that sounds as though scientific doctors have the condition beaten. But in translation 'anorexia nervosa' just means 'not eating for nervous reasons'.

Labels like that are good for scientific medical trade. They serve to make the condition the sole preserve of the scientific medical profession. Yet this need not be the case.

Most orthodox psychiatrists see anorexia as an obsessive dread of fatness; and it is true that weight loss may become an obsessive compulsion leading eventually to death. When it is that severe there is, of course, no option but to involve the doctors.

Bulimia may be associated with it (ancient Greek 'boulimia' = ravenous hunger). Overeating then alternates with vomiting and purging.

The most usual way for scientific medical staff and psychologists to manage eating disorders is to offer positive encouragement and to use persuasive manipulation to maintain nutrition. Just occasionally there may be some attempt to discover reasons why such a destructive pattern of behaviour should have taken hold.

To get out of it and find real healing, however, it is necessary to get into it with your heart. This can be painful. If you will come to Jesus and accept Him as saviour, however, you can humbly allow Holy Spirit to bring relevant issues to light and He will take the pain. Serious difficulties in relationships with familiar people will be discovered. They can be brought to the Lord and healed.

The real presence of Jesus in a person's life makes it possible for truth to be faced and no longer hidden. However, it will often prove impossible for other people who do not know Jesus to understand the truth that will be revealed. Therefore it will be necessary to allow Holy Spirit to bestow shrewdness, so as to know how to act and speak.

An anorexic person may silently be screaming, "I cannot change yet! I will go no further! I cannot conform to your demands! I can swallow no more!" There may be altogether too much unresolved, unfinished business for the person to take any more on board.

You cannot eat with people on whom you feel dependent yet who manipulate you without acknowledging it, who do not really hear you, and who frequently infuriate you, but whom you also want to love. You may feel you owe them all sorts of conflicting obligations. They are your security, particularly when you are feeling weak. This sort of thing builds excruciating conflicts inside you.

You cannot eat with people who turn your deep concerns back on you by accusing you of being mistaken, often through innuendo, whilst denying that they do so. You may understand that they are doing this out of anxiety and ignorance, yet it may seem impossible for them to change because so much depends on their defences being maintained.

Unspeakable dynamics contribute to this dreadful obsession called anorexia nervosa.

So what chance do you have? It seems you cannot win. Whenever there is an opening for you to eat, you overindulge in food in desperation, longing for the comfort it affords. Then you vomit. The situation makes you utterly sick. You may even have a subconscious desire to vomit over them all.

You wilt away with stress. The trauma inflicted on your soul seems as though it will continue until you die.

Although you may forgive the people who contribute to your condition, they may not change. Although you accept Jesus and acknowledge that God is sovereign, and know yourself forgiven by God for reacting with so much self-harm, and although you may have renounced, in the name of Jesus, your bitter hostility, and your anger and hatred and jealousy and stubbornness, and your false guilt and self-rejection and self-hatred and shame, and your crushed spirit and weakness, and a few other matters as well that the Lord will show you, you may still feel stuck. You may need to get away to live somewhere else for a while and recover slowly.

Healing

Getting right with God is the way to healing for all these obsessive conditions. Speaking on a regular basis with someone who understands may assist the process.

Healing the mind usually involves a process that demands perseverance over an extended period of time. Submit yourself to God therefore, and He will reveal in His good timing all that needs to be dealt with.

But it is quite wrong to be passive. It is a terrible mistake to expect Him to do all the work. He has already won the victory for you. Thank God for sending the Lord Jesus and for what He accomplished for you at the cross (Psalm 50:23). Then engage with Him, and be brutally honest with yourself. Bring it all before Him. Be willing to allow and to act on what Holy Spirit reveals.

Forgive those who have sinned against you. Repent of your failings, your sins, and the folly of your reactions, even though you could not avoid them. Order the enemy, in the name of your redeemer Jesus, to stop deceiving you. It may be necessary to resist spirits of confusion and of fear, and to expel them in Jesus' name, and to expel all sorts of other unclean spirits in the same way. The blood of Jesus will wash them out if you belong to Him (see 1 John 1:7 - believe the word of God and it works!). They come out with a cough or a vomit. When you discover the compulsion has gone, you will find God will have healed hidden wounds and deepened your awareness.

DISSOCIATION

Divided from God

It is dreadful to realise that since the Renaissance of Greek and Roman learning nearly a thousand years ago, and the subsequent European Enlightenment, knowledge of spirituality has been steadily supplanted by human invention. Systematic rules of scientific reasoning have become the only commonly accepted means for understanding. Humanism has established its hegemony.

Sadly, most Christians have felt constrained to exult this way of understanding in order to maintain academic respectability and to attract enough people into their institutional buildings for them to remain in religious use. Spiritual knowledge seems to have become more the preserve of pagans than of Christians. But neither pagan spirituality nor humanistic science actually proves sufficient for healing the human soul, whose relationships involve the mind.

Personal relationships are spiritual. Spiritual issues are not just issues of the mind; they are also the concern of real deities who influence people profoundly. Spiritual effects cannot be guaranteed because they are bestowed by a deity not under human control, and their reception depends upon genuine faith and trust. They can never be measured in a way that satisfies secular actuaries who provide money for services. Truthful description is the only way to enable spiritual accounting and gain a measure of their effects.

Consequently, humanistic science does not provide an adequate way of understanding the mind. Under its influence we have become dissociated from God. And God says: *"You turn things upside down, as if the potter were thought to be like the clay! Shall what is formed say to him who formed it, "He did not make me"? Can the pot say of the potter, "He knows nothing"?"* (Isaiah 29:16.)

Practical human inventions, however, do seem to make things better for a while. The systematic scientific use of things to improve the world often seems to be the answer to all our problems. But human nature remains unchanged. Accusations and deceptions not only disturb our peace but can also wreck our minds. And the practical use of substances does not heal mental illness.

True peace, healing and freedom are only found through obedience to the voice of God the Creator of the universe, who is Spirit (John 4:24), who created us in His image (Genesis 1:27), and whose Spirit comes to those who accept His only begotten Son Jesus (John 16:12-15). The answer to humanism is that when the human spirit comes alive in Jesus we really start living with joy. But without the Lord Jesus there is ultimate chaos.

Unredeemed human nature responds to the accusations and deceptions of Satan with pathological censorship which distorts true perception and understanding. We can also be seduced and enchanted, and thereby deceived. In consequence, events fail to be truthfully understood, peace escapes us, and we become separated, dissociated from God who created us.

Censorship

There is a natural physiological mechanism in each one of us for excluding from consciousness whatever seems irrelevant or too much to think about. We are calling it 'the censor'. When the time comes for sleep, it inhibits awareness, causing it to shut down sufficiently. When we are awake it enables us to concentrate on the matter in hand, and it excludes whatever interference might come to mind. We could say that it actively inhibits irrelevance. It serves to protect the heart and mind from engaging with more than they can handle.

When something cannot really be understood, it is tempting to ignore it. This, too, is the operation of the censor. But it might cause us to miss what is important.

It stands to reason that how this natural physiological censor operates will depend upon the system of belief held by the person. What really makes sense according to deeply held belief will tend not to be considered irrelevant, and will not therefore be excluded from consciousness. Thus the censor may be seen to be guided by whoever is truly worshipped.

Everyone holds some principles or ideas to be sacred; and this can easily be seen to be the result of spiritual influence from a spiritual being or deity (even the idea that nothing is sacred and everything is relative can be seen as worship of a deity called the Prince of This World).

Consequently the operation of the censor in a secular person or a pagan will be different from the operation of the censor in a genuine Christian. What seems irrelevant for secular people and people of other faiths may actually be understandable and of relevance for Christians, and vice versa. Different faiths have different priorities, and cause differences in awareness.

Since the God of Israel knows all things (1 John 3:20, Hebrews 4:13), and since those who accept the Lord Jesus as their personal saviour can develop the mind of Christ (1 Corinthians 2:14-16), healing is available for everything ever censored out of a human mind. It is important to know this because in this fallen world the activity of the censor can cause disputes. And putting things out of your mind to try to forget about them is not truly healing.

Shocking events occur and terrible things happen beyond the capacity of the mind immediately to comprehend. Children who are not mature enough to understand properly do not totally dismiss the memory of such events. Nor do adults traumatised by cataclysm or war. Less shocking events, too, can be enduringly disturbing. Behind a good face and a stiff upper lip distressing memories may lie hidden.

Confusion, terror and physical injury stress a person. If turmoil is prolonged, the continual stress weakens both body and mind, so that the censor will come into play more readily in an attempt to protect the person from the shock of further trauma. So people develop irrational fears or there may be subjects to which they are over-sensitive.

When seriously shocking events are too much to take, a state of general inhibition shuts down the mind so that the person may even seem paralysed, in a trance, insensitive to further assault yet hyper-sensitive and hyper-reactive to small stimuli. The person will then be very tense, may not make much sense, and may even run berserk doing crazy things. This sequence of events is seen during continuous bombardment in war, and also in other profoundly stressful circumstances necessitating prolonged, intensive vigilance. The person may be taken into custody and treated. Or the person may eventually collapse from physical exhaustion. The whole system of belief and established habits of mind can totally change during such episodes. The mind can be brainwashed.

Enchantment

We have been created with a capacity to become fascinated and entranced. And when such a state of mind comes upon us there is a partial shut-down and narrowing of conscious awareness as our interest becomes intensely focussed on the object, idea, event or person that has captured and excited our attention. Perception becomes restricted to the experience, putting us in a sort of trance.

A baby suckling at the mother's breast will often fall into a state of partial sleep whilst the baby's awareness of the teat remains focussed enough for the child to suck periodically. During such moments the spirit of the mother affects the child profoundly. Her love blesses her child and encourages her baby to thrive. Eye contact imbues love and assurance. Even if there should be disturbance, the child's sleepy sucking continues under the mother's protection.

When a little older, the child may sit on the mother's knee and fall asleep whilst listening to an enchanting bedtime story. Despite apparently being asleep, the child may not only remember the story but may also be quite deeply affected by it.

Still later in life, an adult can be lulled into the same sort of trance by the soothingly authoritative voice of a hypnotist as the attention of the eyes is focussed, for example, on the hypnotist's finger moving to and fro. The hypnotist can then make suggestions upon which the person will act when fully awake again.

When entranced, the person becomes biddable and willing towards an influence that is trusted. And whether or not an influence is trusted will ultimately depend upon the spiritual system of trust and belief previously inculcated. Even in an entranced state, however, a person will not be willing to betray deepest convictions unless the will is totally broken.

A state of trance can also be produced by violent insecurity and terror, as in war, or by violent spectacle, shock, or induced abandon and frenzy. The trance state then produced will similarly be caused by partial shut-down of awareness by the censor, this time in an attempt to protect the person from overwhelming experience. The experience will be so alarming that constant vigilance is essential. Awareness therefore remains intensely focussed. But terror and violence will open the person to baleful influences, which may remain in the person's soul. The person may even become so lost as to become hopeless. If the disturbance is so severe as to wipe previous conditioning out of the mind, new convictions may become implanted in the mind.

Emotional turmoil induced by violent events, gross misunderstandings, powerful words, powerful music, seductive pictures, spectacular shows, or released through energetic dancing, or hallucinogenic drugs, or even by constant stress, may thus produce a state of insecurity and of trance through which a person may change drastically.

Advertising uses similar psychological knowledge to enrapture and persuade. So do world leaders. Destabilisation sets the stage for change.

People can be manipulated like this without being aware of the truth of what is going on.

Through false worship, and through placing their trust in deceptive ways, the operation of the censor and a state of trance can dissociate us from truth, from God, and from our true selves. Malign influences can pose as wonderful stories and seriously interfere with the plan God has for each one of us, eventually leaving us sick and in pieces.

When people realise this, they may become distressed. Some become hopeless. Some rebel. Others search for God.

The good news is that healing is available through accepting Jesus and repentance.

Personality Disorder and PTSD

Bad experiences naturally cause bad reactions. Cruelty naturally produces fear and hatred. Continuous exposure to disturbance in childhood can obviously cause habitual responses and reflex reactions that are equally disturbing, if not more so. People brought up in unstable environments that naturally produce extreme emotional reactions become habitually disturbing to other people.

If extreme emotional reactions are never tempered with forgiveness, and if unclean spiritual assistance is called upon, knowingly or unknowingly, in an attempt to control distress, demonic spiritual beings may attach themselves to those emotional responses whenever they occur, and from then on those demons may dwell inside the soul. And they will become apparent whenever memory is triggered by any reminder.

Some of those emotional disturbances may have occurred in circumstances so desperate as to be overwhelming. The person is shattered. Some degree of shut-down of conscious awareness of everything but the terror, or the pain, may have produced some degree of trance. Future events that serve as a reminder, in any sort of way, may then threaten to trigger full recall of the original disturbing events. The full memory will be suppressed if it threatens mental breakdown.

Breakdown will be threatened if the censor originally blocked out full awareness of the context, thereby producing confusion instead of understanding. If the individual has never found the space or the necessary help to come to terms with those events, there may be a disturbing acting out of associated emotion in such a way as to afford some relief in current circumstances. This is likely to cause greater confusion and trouble.

This way a person can be driven to be dissociated within their very being, disconnected from wholeness, disturbing to other people, destructive, unpredictable.

Some people who have had many severely bad childhood experiences may even seem to have several different personalities as their thoughts and behaviour automatically adapt to the present company they need to keep. Others become psychopaths, in whom genuine tenderness and kindness are totally prevented by deception.

Disturbing people like this are difficult to live with. Consequently they are said to have a personality disorder.

Healing

There is healing. Understanding is possible with the Lord Jesus. But first it is necessary to recognise that God, the Creator of the universe, is a person, not just an idea. God is sovereign but He is merciful and good, and His love for sinners, and for everything he created, endures for ever. He actually became a human being like us in this world, as His only begotten Son, God with us, in order to save human beings for Himself. This cost His Son, Messiah Jesus, His very lifeblood. He was crucified like a criminal, but He rose from the dead. He has been there. God therefore understands what a mess we are, what impossible situations we find ourselves in, and what pain we have, and He loves us just the same. He even overcame death. He offers us new life and healing.

But we do have to reach out and take hold of Him, and persevere. Therefore come to Him with a humble heart, and continue to thank Him, and praise and worship. Jesus took our sicknesses and pains upon Himself on the cross. He rose from the dead. May His Spirit rest upon you! Resting in Jesus is healing. Allow yourself to follow the process of repentance, forgiveness and healing that He will set before you. With Him, the past can be remembered and healed. It is usually necessary, in God's good timing, actually to realise all that has happened, right back to the beginning, and how it felt. Your demons can be resisted and then expelled by you in Jesus' name. If you need the help of experienced Christians, ask for it.

Hysteria

Occasionally the censor will even shut down a body part, such as an arm, or an eye, if it will serve the purpose of making everything seem sufficiently satisfactory, and at the same time prevent profoundly disturbing memories from coming into consciousness or being acted out.

There is evidence that some acutely stressful emotional (sometimes horrific, sometimes simply powerful) experiences can occasionally cause the mechanism of proprioceptive sensation, which controls our balance, to be shut down. Under spiritual influence (which may or may not be demonic - see 2 Corinthians 12:2-4) this may contribute to being 'slain in the spirit' or to an experience of spiritual (or astral) travelling.

Sometimes acting-out takes over. Examples are sleep-walking, and also so-called fugue states in which a person may suddenly awaken not knowing where they are or how they got there or what has really been going on or even who they are. After some sort of trigger has threatened to re-mind the mind, partial shut-down sometimes needs an element of this sort of acting out in order to keep the person safe from fully remembering what really needs to be faced. Fully remembering will unconsciously threaten to be catastrophic, and the stress of this activates the censor and the partial shut-down.

Hysteria is the medical term for this sort of thing.

Healing may be approached as described above. The root cause needs eventually to be healed and eliminated as a threat by being brought to light with Jesus.

AUTISM

If you are not a genuine Christian there is no point in reading this chapter.

Why?

Because genuine Christians are the only people who know there is healing for guilt. They are the only people who know they are not condemned by it. They are the only people who can handle the feelings of guilt that come naturally through suspecting their own failings may have played some part in hurting their child. They are the only people who know they belong to a human race that is fallen, and who know their Redeemer has paid the price to save them, to heal and to restore. They are the only ones who really know the healing power of His mercy and forgiveness.

The so-called 'autism spectrum' includes Asperger's syndrome. The spectrum is characterised by severe impediments in communication with other people, stressful obsessiveness and a gross lack of natural empathy.

Autistic people seem to live in a world of their own. Extreme autism is characterised by isolated withdrawal into oneself, obsessive relationships with objects and order rather than with people, not hearing almost as if deaf, difficulty with abstract concepts, impoverished expression (language, writing), use of repetitive phrases that have been heard from other people, an overriding need to avoid change, aggressive reactions to interference, antisocial reactions and even self-harm. There are various degrees of severity. But a good percentage of those so afflicted respond well to the sort of specialised help that involves genuine kindness and empathetic interest in the experience of the autistic person.

The condition continues to be subject to scientific investigation. Genetic studies cannot offer much explanation. There is some evidence that synaptic dysfunction may have developed at certain nerve endings in the brain during early stages of pregnancy. But science has discovered no definite unifying mechanism for the condition.

Some of the parents of those afflicted have been said to have been rather cold and formal individuals, the sort of people who have become unemotional and constantly concerned with abstractions, not the sort spontaneously to wear their hearts on their sleeves. Parental homes of the people whom I have known to have been diagnosed as autistic have all been subtly stressful, due to the impossibility (for various reasons) of expressing natural emotional responses. During pregnancy with the child who turned out to be autistic there was constant fear, constant threat of violence, or in some cases, the most dreadful worry, coupled with a desperate need to keep up appearances. Such stress keeps you on edge, and can prevent a person (in this case, perhaps, the baby) from hearing and perceiving.

Because of the block on insinuating guilt there has been virtually no scientific research on the nature of the instinctive communication between the mother and the baby in her womb. There is a lack of understanding of the effect of a mother's emotional state on her unborn child.

It does seem as though maternal stress may pass through the placental barrier and affect the developing child in the early months of pregnancy.

If a mother's excessive emotional stress during early pregnancy should be the cause of autism, however, I am sure the Lord can heal it. I am sure that if the face of God is sought in the name of Jesus Christ, His Son, God will heal both the physical damage and the unclean spirits in the person afflicted, which may turn out to have been associated with stressful events that afflicted the mother during her pregnancy.

When mothers communicate with children in their wombs, they would be wise to communicate with God as well, and pray for the children they carry, and seek God's protection, peace and guidance.

PSYCHOSIS

Mania

People become so some extent manic when they flee. When escaping terror or death, desperate measures are taken. Search for safety takes priority over everything else. Stress is high. The censor restricts the focus. There is no time to be bothered with sensibilities.

The threat may be an emergency in the external world, such as accident, attack, fire or catastrophe. Or the threat may arise from the internal world.

Threats may appear from the internal world by a reminder that threatens to trigger memory of excruciating, old, unhealed wounds that lie hidden in the unconscious. Opening up that sort of thing can sometimes threaten breakdown of all ability to cope. When a person is fleeing from such internal pain, their behaviour may cause a great deal of concern to others.

The original events that caused internally suppressed pain will probably be from childhood before the age of eight. Because children are usually dependent upon, or at least trusting towards, those who cause their pain, and because they lack sufficient maturity fully to understand and to resolve difficult situations, their memory of stressful childhood events is often confused, and often remains unhealed.

But the pain will not only be from childhood. Something will have occurred in the present, the dynamics of which are similar to excruciating events buried in unconscious memory from childhood. When there is urgency without any apparent possibility of coming to terms with the details of what is going on, or of finding any peace, the impulse to flee may take over in desperation. Desperate flight may then become desperately irresponsible.

Mania arises in apparently-enforced denial of confusion, shock, horror, agony and pain. Psychotic mania is a state of being wildly and demonically driven into carefree elation, excitement, over-activity, sleeplessness, over-confidence, loss of usual inhibitions, and grossly inappropriate behaviour. Demonic spirits of terror, pride and lust, and so on, may attach themselves to the crazy behaviour and induce grandiose delusions, with hallucinations, excitable and grossly irresponsible activity, and incomprehensible babbling. An afflicted individual may spend money unreservedly, and become the most appalling nuisance, utterly headstrong, unwilling to allow any mutual understanding with anyone else. It proves totally impossible to reason with the person. And it becomes imperative to stop further violence. This is generally considered to be a medical emergency. Powerful sedation becomes the only solution.

If a degree of mania or hypomania alternates on a fairly regularly basis with depression, it is called a **bipolar** affective disorder. In this case the same sort of internal confusion and pain is also causing depressions. Periodic episodes of fleeing from the confusion and pain alternate with suffering the wretched misery of searching internally to come to terms with it.

Frenzy is a rather more controlled sort of mania. Frenzy can be whipped up by excitement, by drug induced thrills and by demonic influences. Stress plays a big part. Both physical excitement and powerful emotions are stressful, and they can be generated artificially in order to induce frenzy. Constant stress weakens resilience and exacerbates frenzied desperation. People can be manipulated this way to demonstrate, or to be violent.

We should remember, too, that very serious danger in the present can also cause extraordinarily crazy behaviour. We see it sometimes after catastrophic events. Perhaps the most poignant example ever known was the dancing mania that took hold of groups of people all over Europe who were terrified of the Black Death, which rapidly halved the population in the fourteenth century.

Healing for all forms of mania, including psychotic mania, involves facing the root cause, the original confusion and pain, or the original event or mistake, or whatever it was, and bringing it to the cross of Jesus, for He took our pains. We can only truly face things like this with Jesus. He actually knows about it all (Hebrews 4:13). He will reveal the true facts, showing us no more than we can take at any one time (1 Corinthians 10:13). He was there and it is by the grace of God that we survive.

Healing involves forgiving other people, and accepting forgiveness from God for all the natural reactions and mistakes of the fallen human nature of all concerned, because we accept that Jesus paid the price with His lifeblood to redeem us from our sin (Ephesians 1:7). It involves saying "Thank you" to Him continually, for our pains and sicknesses do not usually depart all at once. Indeed, it is often a battle between fighting off doubt from Satan and accepting and trusting what the word of God says in Isaiah 53:4: *"Surely He has borne our illnesses and carried our pains."* (TLV.)

It usually takes time. Most people feel unable to face the root causes all at once. They will talk all around the subject. Experience indicates the necessity of patiently allowing them to do so. Sometimes people cannot even believe what they said when they finally tell the Lord the really pertinent facts. But once the root cause comes to light in the Lord's presence, true healing will have begun.

Schizophrenia

Although the odd attitudes and behaviour called schizophrenia could start at any time in adult life, most frequently it appears first in the late teens or in the twenties after leaving home, whilst attempting to engage with a different culture. Being cursed and rejected are often what initially precipitate confusion and delusion.

Heart, mind and soul may be found to have failed to acquire sufficient stability and maturity to allow the individual to be flexible enough to handle offence, and to adapt to new territory. The securities of perception and belief to which the person was hitherto accustomed seem not have been grounded in sufficiently sound spiritual truth to cope with the challenges of the new environment.

So although the trouble commonly manifests in early adulthood, the root of the trouble lies in childhood.

The very word schizophrenia is derived from ancient Greek words that imply a tendency to division of heart and mind; and an afflicted individual can be seen not only to have suddenly become separated from God and from ordinary society, but also to have become divided up within, suddenly lacking integrity of spirit and soul. Insecurity, wrong conclusions and crazy behaviour take over their very being.

Most schizophrenic people will have been living for a long time with hidden stress. Then come destabilisation and breakdown, suddenly causing horrendous disturbance to close relatives.

The schizophrenic person will doubt other people's apparent intentions, or ignore them, or misperceive, or believe delusions and act on them. Preoccupation with hallucinations may further isolate the individual. Acting on the direction of hallucinatory voices may sometimes be dangerous. Powerfully frustrated emotions may make behaviour chaotic, irresponsible and unpredictable. Speech may be incoherent and jumbled. Sometimes mannerisms, or attitudes and postures, may be adopted for long periods. There may be a strange paranoia. There may be stupor. There may be gross over-activity.

Under profound but hidden stress, the censorship mechanism will have closed down at random, in confusion, and the person may be seen rapidly to have become open to deception by all sorts of influences, ideas and powerful spirits.

Behaviour can quickly become utterly intolerable. One can feel constantly pounded and dreadfully weakened by spending too long in the company of someone flagrantly psychotic. It soon becomes entirely natural to want them to be controlled and shut away.

Sometimes, however, it is possible for a personal relationship to develop that calms things down and holds them enough for true sense to begin to return. Although sudden healings have occurred, more commonly it takes a considerable period of time for adequate interpersonal contact to be made so that the many contributory factors can be laid bare and healed.

Medical attention

If the psychosis comes to medical attention the individual will probably be treated with powerful, sedative drugs which subdue the thinking and slur the speech, and which may cause dryness of the mouth and shakiness, or sometimes distorted body movements. Many such people are locked away in psychiatric units guarded by secular custodians, out of contact with everyday humanity and difficult to visit. A denied but oppressive and pervasive hopelessness and meaninglessness may readily be discerned in such places.

The medical profession classifies schizophrenia according to its prevailing manifestations, which differ from person to person. They diagnose, classify and treat according to objective criteria.

But some sedation may be constructively used, either constantly or intermittently, to hold the person and prevent damage from crazy behaviour whilst progress is made in accountability. If the dose befuddles the mind it will be counterproductive. But used responsibly with the person's compliance, it will sometimes usefully assist healing.

Insecurity and alienation

These, then, easily become banished people, rejected, cursed and sent outside the city gate. But they are people whom Jesus is inviting to the great banquet (Luke 14:23-24, Hebrews 13:13). Of course, they cannot be forced to come. They do, however, need an opportunity to re-connect with human beings, as well as with God. Disciples of the Lord Jesus who carry the Spirit of eternal truth are better equipped to meet them than professional secular custodians. The love and truth of God are healing.

Personal contact must be made for the process of healing to begin. And during the process of healing, all sorts of diverse issues and dynamics will be found to have contributed during childhood to undermining the wholeness and security of heart and mind, thereby generating the schizophrenia. Curses in particular, sometimes generational curses, will be found to have played a significant part.

Despite having grown up with a profound insecurity, the child's world will have held together well enough until new challenges became too difficult later on. Despite feeling broken up inside, it will probably have remained possible to put on the good face demanded by the family whilst living at 'home'. Trouble will have come with the challenges of a different environment where that good face is no longer sufficient.

How schizophrenia may develop

A young child is vulnerable, and dependent upon parents. Parents are believed. Sense develops out of earliest relationships. Those relationships, therefore, need to be good enough, credible enough, stable enough, loving and truthful enough. These are godly qualities, and when we say we human beings are created by God in His image we are acknowledging that when we love God with all our heart and mind and strength and love our neighbours as ourselves those qualities bring a sound foundation into heart and mind and soul and enable sound maturity to develop. Mankind responds well to God's goodness, truth and justice as expressed in Holy Scripture (Romans 3:4 KJV or TLV). No parent is perfect, but there needs to be enough of all this, and parents do need to be good enough. And it is hard to accept that sometimes they may not be, and their ancestors may not have been, although none of them may actually be culpable, for they may not have been able to help it. We all belong to a human race that is fallen. Yet all can be healed in Jesus.

False religion and false worship by parents and ancestors may be the cause of conflicts and insecurities in the soul that make the person less capable of adapting to any change of culture, and less able to understand the change. It is who is worshipped that provides the basic security of any culture. Failure to heed the God of Israel undermines basic security (Deuteronomy 28:28).

Stress in a child may also be caused by the people the child believes in not being sure in themselves that they mean what they say. Meaning is then sensed to be inauthentic. The child automatically picks up the ambivalence. Hereditary insecurity in a parent may thus be transmitted to the child. Quite often there is a discernible hereditary element in the genesis of schizophrenia.

Overt hypocrisy in parents may be more intentional. If religion is propounded through rules, for example, without real relationship with the spiritual being who is worshipped, it leaves room for people to be actors and hypocrites. If obedience is imposed by rules, it can be inculcated with stress, preventing sound knowledge being the fruit of love. The child will be aware of this. It becomes possible to be religiously acceptable simply by obeying the rules, without believing and trusting the one in whom faith is professed (2 Timothy 3:5 refers). The child may then be confounded by being insistently told that things are as the rules would have it, whilst the child's actual experience is that this is not the case. Yet the child's experience is denied, and the child can consequently be seriously rejected for expressing it. Those in whom the child believes may thus chronically deny the facts of the child's experience and refuse to engage with it, which can seriously undermine the child's confidence in perception.

Hypocrisy often hides unacknowledged guilt, and parental attempts to make reparation for guilt can seem to the child like strange behaviour that defeats understanding. This sort of thing, too, will affect the child, even if only subliminally, and undermine the child's security.

If the child's alleged experience is denied by the parents, the child will be disconcerted. If such denial persists, the child may react either in a passive way, accepting that there are secrets that should never be spoken about, and expecting that there is nothing for it but to have a secret life separate from others; or the child may react in an aggressive way with overt rebellion. Or there may be a mixture of both. If those secrets involve abuse of the child, or illegal activities, or threats of violence, the child's repressed reactions may be extreme, yet the original details will remain hidden, and associated reactions will only be revealed if a threat appears that could trigger the memory. Abusive childhood shocks that have never been healed will contribute to the shattering of fundamental, inner, personal security. Rebellion may turn to rage and rage can turn to madness. Hallucinogenic drug abuse will make it worse. The rebellion may even be encouraged and developed by families interested to make their children agents of destructive opposition to Christianity, or other religions, or civilisations.

Blame and rejection, and being roundly cursed by other people, may readily follow. Terror may then set in to further break up the inner being. Such reactions will usually be repressed. If the person becomes conscious of them, however, those natural reactions can rapidly be overwhelming. As a result, the child may feel 'all in pieces' inside yet able to put on a good face, but prone suddenly to manifest very distressing behaviour. The child may even grow up seeming to have several different personalities, because different aspects of the feelings and thoughts that have been repressed need to be hidden in different situations.

Whatever cannot be made sense of sufficiently to bring real peace is naturally dumped into memory which is unspeakable, held secretly in the dark, in the 'unconscious', where confusion continues to cause stress, and from where trouble can rear its head if triggered. Dreams and imaginings and various adventures are nevertheless influenced by this material in the unconscious, contributing to delusion and false conclusions. Too much of this unresolved material, too much hidden confusion and falsehood, undermines one's inner security, and can make a person crazy, or sometime physically ill.

Essentially, it is whatever builds overriding insecurity, fear, rage, rejection and confusion into a child before the age of about eight that may predispose to psychotic schizophrenic breakdown in later years.

Feelings and thoughts, which are repressed natural responses to actual past events, will have been embellished subsequently by what the person has made of their experiences. If the person's secret world is allowed to flood the mind, it can threaten to be overwhelming. To some extent the threat may be projected into the outside environment (which is most notable in paranoid schizophrenia) and to some extent this is usually justified because the social environment will impose severe sanctions on unacceptable behaviour. So other people may seem threatening. This increases stress, and the stress becomes chronic. Unclean spirits get in. The stress contributes to hallucinatory experience. Voices are believed. Delusions set in. Behaviour and thought become so erratic that they cannot adequately be communicated. Language becomes garbled. It seems as though no one understands. Social exclusion begets a sense of rejection. It may also beget stubborn hatred of the whole world. Sometimes people react with total defeat and passive hopelessness. Some afflicted individuals celebrate their oddity with pride. They may even assume obnoxious delusions of control. Cursing and rejection from other people are often the final factor that leads to hospitalisation. Then hospitalisation leads to heavy medication.

Decisions about what to do with the disturbing person are often taken without totally open consultation with the person involved, and without the person involved being allowed to be aware of the real intentions, thoughts and feelings of other people concerned. So the disturbing person will naturally be further confused and feel manipulated, which in turn may generate anger, stubbornness and hopelessness. When no-one will believe them, and they can do nothing but comply with overriding authority, their will is stultified or broken. It can seem like a death to them. The desires of the heart become influenced by unclean spirits. They readily become wretchedly unpredictable.

Healing

"Since the children have flesh and blood, He too shared in their humanity so that by His death He might destroy him who holds the power of death – that is, the devil – and free those who all their lives were held in slavery by their fear of death." (Hebrews 2:14-15.)

God loves us and never takes away our free will. He wants our relationship with Him to be freely given whilst He equips us to meet the fallen world in truth. In a person who has lapsed into schizophrenia, therefore, the heart and the will both need healing so that they become free of all that gets in the way. Healing the mind follows.

A safe place is needed. The ambience should be conducive to reflection. Even though the will may be stultified or broken, a person's heart remains their own. Healing comes through being closely involved with other people through whom the Spirit of truth begins to touch the heart. Straightforward, empathetic personal contact is necessary in order to break through the deadness and convey sound sense. Legalistic and theoretical words, and good advice, will not really register.

The prayers of other people of true faith certainly help. The battle for sanity is spiritual. Schizophrenic people are trapped in unwitting collusion with the spiritual forces of this fallen world. The subtle accusations and deceptions of the prince of this world were overcome by Jesus, the Son of God, at the cross, and those who accept the price Jesus paid for our redemption are invited to appropriate God's spiritual gifts in order to defeat the enemy with the sword of Holy Spirit. Spiritual authority is given to true disciples of Jesus, as in Matthew 10:1, and it will be called upon. The binding and loosing of spiritual powers, as in Matthew 16:19, may be needed at a moment's notice. Those involved must therefore stay right with God, be self-controlled and fit, and be versed in spiritual warfare.

It can be of great help to give careful, regular, empathetic attention to afflicted individuals over a lengthy period of time, and to keep faith with them. Furthermore, groups of people who have had similar experiences can be wisely refereed and encouraged to assist each other in making sense of events. Sharing eases the very considerable pain.

It should be carefully noted, however, that fear of litigation in multicultural societies (consequent upon different ways of understanding) means this sort of assistance for schizophrenic people is never funded by the state. It has generally become impossible for Christians to have this sort of relationship with schizophrenic people in psychiatric facilities whilst at the same time keeping their spiritual integrity.

Those of God's people with an interest in healing will probably need to stand with the person said to have schizophrenia against the judgements of the world, and commonly against the opinions of the family, too. The culture and relationships of the early environment within the family will have provided a pattern of control the person unwittingly continues to seek for security. Not only will the family commonly endeavour to maintain those controls, but the schizophrenic person will often be found to expect other people, too, to exert those controls. Others will be assumed to think and behave like family members did in days gone by. But this can be a hindrance to healing, because the schizophrenic person seeking freedom in Jesus will also be being quietly encouraged by Holy Spirit to break free and get strong enough to carry his or her own load with a mind of their own (Galatians 6:5).

It is instructive and encouraging to see that Jesus Himself had to deal with similar issues in His own family. In Mark 3:21 (TLV) we find His family going to take charge of Him, saying *"He's out of His mind!"* But in verses 32 to 35 we read: *"A crowd was sitting around Him, and they tell Him, "Look, Your mother and Your brothers are outside looking for You." Answering them, He said, "Who are My mother and My brothers?" Looking at those sitting in a circle around Him, He said, "Here are My mother and My brothers! For whoever does the will of God, he is My brother and sister and mother.""* Later, of course, His family became reconciled to Him.

Those involved with someone schizophrenic, however, will need to hear what the person is really saying, so that truth may be mutually discerned amidst powerful emotions, confusion and distorted thinking. Getting to the truth with people caught in this world can be turbulent, particularly if there should be rebellion against old family controls that come to be seen, in the course of time, to have been dominating, intimidating and inauthentic. As Jesus is taken hold of, however, and as His light and truth pervade perception, the person breaks out into new territory and is able to forgive, and to be forgiven. Letting go of the old and coming into the new can be a remarkable experience. The person's mind is restored so that they have a mind of their own, freely to be in accord with the mind of God. As both this fallen world and also the kingdom of God are seen in the light of truth through Jesus, the heart and the will are brought alive to become the firm foundation for soundness of mind.

Jesus' claim to be the way, the truth and the life (John 14:6) proves true. He is the way out of pain, rejection, sickness and torment. Truth comes through knowing Him through His Spirit living in your heart. He heals the mind in accordance with Scripture. He takes all the shame. He breaks the curse. His presence heals confusion. Through telling Him the pain, new life is found in Him.

Appealing to Jesus, however, must definitely involve a humble heart. Desperation, pride, fury, self-pity, resentment, and stress, will prevent a person hearing and responding to Him (Deuteronomy 28:15 & 28). If that sort of thing persists, terror will supervene (Deuteronomy 28:66).

How such devastation has arisen needs to be reflected upon with a humble heart and a willingness to forgive and be forgiven. The afflicted person must not remain adamant and proud, but must come to the Lord in repentance and faith. Powerful emotions, which may surface as the past begins to make true sense, must be confessed as sin before Him, and His mercy accepted. So must delusion, when its nature becomes apparent. Delusions and hallucinations respond to testing the spirits, as in 1 John 4:1.

God is sovereign. Our demons will flee after we submit to Him and then resist them in Jesus' name (James 4:7).

Once more, and finally

God says, *"Be still and know that I am God."* (Psalm 46:10.)

The way of healing for the mind is like this:-

- get to know the Lord Jesus Christ, God made flesh, born of a virgin, God's "only begotten Son" who was crucified but overcame death and rose from the grave;
- accept that He shared our humanity on this earth and knows absolutely everything about each one of us (Hebrews 2:14-18, 4:13 and 1 John 3:20) and can empathise with it;
- accept His love;
- come to Him with a humble heart;
- through Him, allow truth to dawn (but not as the world sees);
- see truly and face pain with Him;
- accept His redeeming sacrifice of Himself on the cross for each one of us, and give thanks, and praise Him and offer Him worship;

- humble your heart and be willing to forgive;
- repent - admit that your fallen human nature has led you into so very many mistakes, and confess them all as sin;
- forgive all those who have sinned against you;
- renounce your sinful ways, and expel any demons in the name of Jesus - cough them out;
- accept the forgiveness and healing freely offered by almighty God because you have accepted Jesus Christ as your saviour;
- then thank God, praise Him and worship Him.

Healing the mind is frequently a process that takes perseverance and endurance. The process described here will probably need to be repeated.

Those of us who choose to accept with grateful hearts the price Jesus Christ paid for us have the option of allowing His Holy Spirit to transform our minds and our lives for a significant place in His eternal kingdom. Our place will be determined by the character formed in us by God's grace as we persevere through this world.

Jesus is coming back soon to reign on this earth and those He has redeemed and equipped will be with Him, and will reign with Him for ever. This applies to people who have suffered mental illness as much as to anyone else.

CORROBORATION

H. Wheeler Robinson (1911) *"The Christian Doctrine of Man"* Edinburgh, T. & T. Clark.

Aubrey R. Johnson (1949) *"The Vitality of the Individual in the Thought of Ancient Israel"* Cardiff, University of Wales Press.

C. Ryder Smith (1951) *"The Bible Doctrine of Man"* London, Epworth Press.

Derek Prince (1915-2003) *"Blessing or Curse - You Can Choose"* and *"They Shall Expel Demons"*- and all Derek Prince's work, which is available through Derek Prince Ministries.

The Book of Common Prayer (1662) *"The Order for the Visitation of the Sick"* and *"The Communion of the Sick"*.

Ruth Hawkey (1996) *"Healing the Human Spirit"* Chichester, New Wine Press. ISBN 1-874367-45-0.

Henry W. Wright (2019) *"Be in Health a More Excellent Way"* Thomaston, Pleasant Valley Publications.

A. T. Boisen (1936) *"The Exploration of the Inner World"* Philadelphia, University of Philadelphia Press, 1971.

Dr. Denis V. Martin (1962) *"Adventure in Psychiatry"* Oxford, Bruno Cassirer.

Søren Kierkegaard (1844) *"The Concept of Anxiety".*

Georg W. Groddeck (1923) *"The Book of the It"* translated by V.M.E. Collins, M.A., London, Vision Press, 1949.

Sigmund Freud (1896) *"The Aetiology of Hysteria"* - James Strachey's translation reprinted in Jeffrey Masson (1984) *"The Assault on Truth"* London, Fontana, 1992.

Robert N. Rapoport (1960) *"Community as Doctor"* London, Tavistock Publications.

R. D. Laing and A. Esterson (1964) *"Sanity, Madness and the Family"* London, Tavistock Publications.

Ivan P. Pavlov (1927) *"Lectures on Conditioned Reflexes: Volume 2, Conditioned Reflexes and Psychiatry"* Translated by Horsley Gantt, London, Lawrence & Wishart, 1941.

Professor Gordon Turnbull (2011) *"Trauma"* London, Transworld Publishers (Corgi - Bantam Press).

Gregory Bateson, D. D. Haley, J. Weakland (1956) *"Towards a Theory of Schizophrenia"* Behavioural Science, Volume 1, Number 4, also published in Gregory Bateson *"Steps to an Ecology of Mind"* St Albans, Paladin, 1973.

John Gordon (2019) *"Healing Madness"*, and *"Get Real"* Edinburgh, Philadelphia Books. ISBNs 978-0-9570970-9-4 and 978-0-9570970-8-7. Available on Amazon.

Printed in Great Britain
by Amazon

87033180R00068